CW01648583

TRIUMPH OVER EMOTIONAL EATING

HOW ANYONE CAN QUICKLY IDENTIFY & MANAGE TRIGGERS, OVERCOME THE SHAME OF BINGEING, COMBAT BODY IMAGE ISSUES, & TRANSFORM THEIR RELATIONSHIP WITH FOOD

LAWRENCE E. MEADOWS

© **Copyright Lawrence E. Meadows/ Michawell LLC, 2024. All rights reserved.**

Legal Notice:

This book is copyright protected and is only for personal use. You cannot amend, distribute, sell, use, quote or paraphrase any part of the content within this book, without the consent of the author or publisher.

Disclaimer Notice:

Please note the information contained within this document is for educational and entertainment purposes only. All effort has been expended to present accurate, up-to-date, and reliable, complete information. No warranties of any kind are declared or implied. Readers acknowledge that the author is not engaging in the rendering of legal, financial, or professional advice.

The information is not intended as medical advice. The content is not a substitute for professional medical care, diagnosis, or treatment. Always seek the advice of your physician or other qualified healthcare provider with any questions you may have regarding a medical or psychiatric condition. Please consult a licensed professional before attempting any techniques outlined in this book. The content within this book has been derived from various sources.

In this book, the names of individuals have been changed to protect their privacy. Any resemblance to actual persons is purely coincidental. The stories and examples presented are based on real experiences but have been altered to ensure confidentiality and respect the privacy of those involved. Any identifying details have been modified to maintain anonymity.

By reading this document, the reader agrees that under no circumstances is the author responsible for any losses, direct or indirect, which are incurred as a result of the use of the information contained within this document, including (but not limited to) errors, omissions, or inaccuracies.

CONTENTS

INTRODUCTION

One evening, I found myself standing in front of the kitchen pantry, the door wide open, staring blankly at shelves stocked with cookies and chocolate bars. My day had been rough, filled with stress and frustration, and all I could think about was finding comfort in these familiar snacks. Before I knew it, I was sitting on the couch, surrounded by empty wrappers, feeling a mix of guilt, shame, and confusion. This wasn't the first time I had turned to food for solace, and I knew it wouldn't be the last unless something changed.

You're not alone in this struggle. Emotional eating is a challenge faced by many, often silently. In the United States, it's estimated that nearly 30% of adults engage in emotional eating. That staggering statistic highlights just how common this issue is. Yet, despite its prevalence, emotional eating often remains shrouded in secrecy and shame.

So, what exactly is emotional eating? At its core, emotional eating is when you use food to cope with your emotions rather than to satisfy physical hunger. It's reaching for that tub of ice cream after a tough day at work or munching on a bag of chips when you're feeling lonely. Emotional eating is a way to numb or avoid unpleasant feelings, but it often leads to a cycle of guilt and further emotional distress.

I'm passionate about this topic and believe I can help you. I've experienced firsthand the deep-seated shame and frustration that comes with bingeing, the constant battle with body image issues, and the desperate desire to find a healthier relationship with food.

The purpose of this book is simple: to provide you with the tools and insights you need to overcome emotional eating. Together, we'll explore practical strategies to identify and manage your triggers, develop mindful eating habits, and cultivate self-compassion. You'll find emotional support and encouragement throughout these pages because healing from emotional eating is not just about changing your eating habits but also about nurturing your mental and emotional well-being.

The impact of emotional eating goes beyond just weight gain or loss. Emotional eating can take a toll on your mental and emotional health, leading to feelings of guilt, shame, and low self-esteem. Physically, it can contribute to health problems like obesity, diabetes, and heart disease. By tackling this issue head-on, you can improve your overall well-being and find more balance and happiness.

This book is structured to guide you step-by-step on this journey. In the first few chapters, we'll focus on understanding emotional eating and identifying your personal triggers. We'll then move on to building healthier coping strategies and practicing mindful eating. You'll learn about the importance of self-compassion and how to foster a positive body image. We'll also delve into the societal influences that shape our connection with food and how to navigate them.

Throughout the book, you'll find a compassionate, nonjudgmental tone. This is a safe space for you to explore your emotions and habits without fear of criticism. The goal is to support you, help you feel understood and validated, and provide practical advice that you can apply in your daily life.

I encourage you to actively engage with the content. Reflect on your experiences, practice the exercises, and apply the strategies discussed. You'll find interactive elements such as journaling prompts and practical exercises designed to deepen your understanding and facilitate growth.

Change is possible. It won't always be easy, and there will be setbacks, but every small, consistent step you take will lead to significant, lasting improvements. Approach this journey with hope and determination and remember that you are not alone. Together, we can triumph over emotional eating!

CHAPTER 1
UNDERSTANDING EMOTIONAL EATING

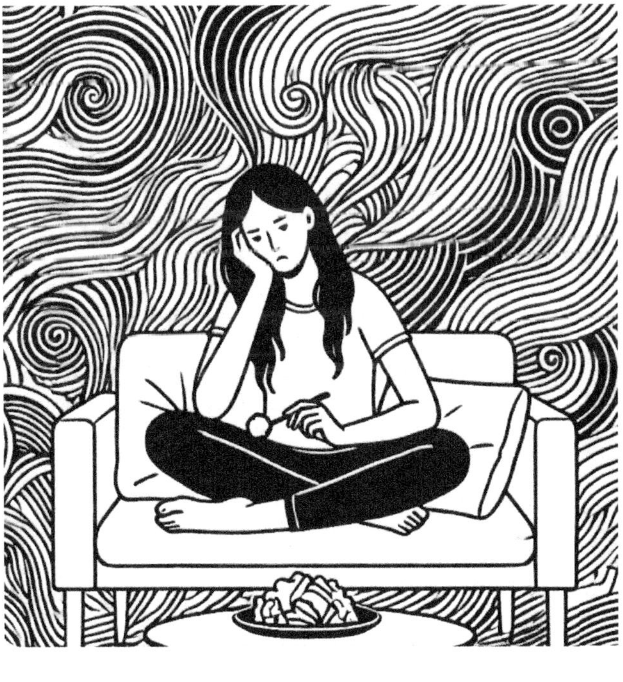

Emotional eating is a term that might sound familiar, yet it holds different meanings for different people. At its core, emotional eating means using food to manage your emotions rather than to satisfy physical hunger. It's not about the occasional indulgence or the joy of savoring a delicious meal; it's about eating to cope with stress, anxiety, sadness, or even boredom. Understanding emotional eating is the first step to overcoming it, and this chapter aims to shed light on what it truly means.

DEFINING EMOTIONAL EATING: WHAT IT IS AND WHAT IT ISN'T

Emotional eating is when you turn to food not because your body needs fuel but because your mind seeks comfort or distraction. It's like using food as a temporary bandage for your emotions.

One of the most critical aspects of emotional eating is understanding the difference between emotional and physical hunger.

- Physical hunger is your body's way of telling you it needs nourishment. It builds gradually, can be satisfied with a variety of foods, and stops once you're full.
- Emotional hunger, on the other hand, comes on suddenly and often craves specific comfort foods. It doesn't stem from a physical need but from an emotional one, and it often leads to eating mindlessly, without satisfaction.

Emotional eating often serves as a coping mechanism. When you feel stressed, bored, lonely, or sad, food can become a way to numb or escape those emotions, even if only temporarily. It provides a quick fix and momentary relief but doesn't address the underlying issue.

It's crucial to dispel some common misconceptions about emotional eating. One of the biggest myths is that emotional eating is simply a lack of willpower. This couldn't be further from the truth. Emotional eating is a complex behavior influenced by a multitude of factors, including emotional, psychological, and environmental triggers. It's not about being weak or undisciplined; it's about how you've learned to cope with your emotions.

Another misconception is that emotional eating means you have a severe eating disorder. While emotional eating can be a component of more serious eating disorders, it doesn't necessarily mean you have one. It's a behavior that many people experience at different levels and for various reasons. Understanding this can help reduce the stigma and shame often associated with emotional eating.

Furthermore, it's also essential to differentiate between emotional eating and binge eating disorder. While they can overlap, they are not the same. Binge eating disorder is characterized by episodes of eating large quantities of food in a short period, often accompanied by a feeling of loss of control. Emotional eating, on the other hand, may not always involve large quantities of food or a sense of loss of control. It's more about the emotional reasons behind why you're eating.

When you recognize and define emotional eating, you start to see how it fits into your life. In those moments, you turn to food for reasons other than hunger, seeking a distraction. It's not about blaming yourself or feeling ashamed; it's about understanding a behavior many people experience and finding healthier avenues to cope with your emotions.

THE PSYCHOLOGY AND BRAIN CHEMISTRY BEHIND EMOTIONAL EATING: WHY WE TURN TO FOOD

Understanding why we reach for that extra slice of pizza often starts with recognizing our psychological triggers. Stress is one of the biggest culprits. When you encounter stressful situations, your body releases cortisol, the "stress hormone." Cortisol prepares your body to fight or flee. However, it can also increase your appetite, particularly for high-fat and sugary foods. Cortisol pushes you to seek out quick energy sources to cope with stress.

But it's not just stress; emotional eating often stems from a need to regulate emotions. Food can be a temporary balm for sadness, loneliness, or boredom. When you eat, your brain releases dopamine, a neurotransmitter associated with pleasure and reward. This dopamine rush can make you feel better, albeit temporarily. It's a quick fix but doesn't solve the underlying emotional issues. Certain foods (you guessed it, high-fat and sugary foods) cause your brain to release dopamine. This makes you feel good and reinforces the behavior, encouraging you to eat those foods again. It's a cycle that can be hard to break.

Serotonin, another neurotransmitter, is key to mood regulation. Low serotonin levels are linked to feelings of depression and anxiety. Interestingly, carbohydrates can temporarily boost serotonin levels, so you might crave bread or pasta when feeling down.

The connection between food and the brain's pleasure centers is profound. Eating activates the brain's reward pathways, creating a sense of pleasure and satisfaction. This is why comfort foods are aptly named—they bring comfort by activating these pleasure centers. This connection can make breaking the emotional eating habit difficult because your brain has learned to associate food with emotional relief.

Furthermore, past trauma can also play a significant role in emotional eating. People who have experienced trauma often use food as a coping mechanism. It's a way to find comfort and a sense of control in an unpredictable world. Emotional eating becomes a form of self-soothing. For instance, someone who experienced neglect during childhood might turn to food as a source of reliable comfort, filling an emotional void that was never addressed. This habit can persist into adulthood, manifesting as emotional eating whenever they feel insecure or stressed.

Various mental health conditions like anxiety, depression, and ADHD can also be associated with emotional eating. Anxiety can make you feel a constant sense of unease, leading you to seek comfort in food. Depression often brings about feelings of hopelessness or sadness, which can make food seem like a way to alleviate those feelings, even if just for a moment. ADHD, with its challenges in impulse control, can make it difficult to stick to regular eating habits, often leading to bingeing episodes as a way to manage emotional dysregulation.

Psychological theories offer more insights into emotional eating. For instance, Maslow's hierarchy of needs suggests that when basic needs like emotional security and self-esteem are unmet, people turn to other sources, like food, for comfort. Food can become a stand-in for the emotional nourishment you lack if you're feeling unfulfilled in your relationships or career.

Moreover, childhood experiences also play a critical role. Attachment theory postulates that early relationships with caregivers shape how you handle stress and emotions later in life. If you were comforted with food as a child, you might continue to seek comfort in food as an adult during stressful times.

Clinical psychologists often point out that emotional eating is a learned behavior that can be unlearned with the right strategies and support. Dr. Jane Smith, a renowned psychologist, states "Emotional eating is not about the food itself but about the emotions that drive the behavior. Addressing those emotions is key to overcoming emotional eating."

Understanding the psychological and chemical factors behind emotional eating can help you understand your habits. It is essential to recognize the intricate web of stress, emotions, past experiences, and brain chemistry that influence your relationship with food. By acknowledging the contribution of these factors, you can begin to address the root causes of emotional eating, paving the way for healthier coping mechanisms and a better relationship with food.

THE CYCLE OF EMOTIONAL EATING: RECOGNIZING THE VICIOUS LOOP

Emotional eating often begins with a triggering event. It might be a fight with a loved one or even just feeling restlessness. This trigger sets off a cascade of emotions that feel overwhelming. To manage these emotions, you may turn to food for comfort. This response is not about hunger but about finding a quick way to soothe those uncomfortable feelings. Imagine coming home after a bad day. You feel frustrated and anxious. Instead of addressing these emotions head-on, you reach for junk food. Eating provides a temporary escape, a way to dull the emotional pain.

After indulging in emotional eating, you might experience a brief moment of relief. The food has served its purpose, offering a fleeting sense of comfort. However, this relief is soon overshadowed by feelings of guilt. You start to criticize yourself for overeating and for not having more self-control. These negative emotions can be just as distressing as the original trigger, if not more so. This self-criticism reinforces the idea that you are somehow "failing," which only adds to your emotional burden. It's a paradox: eating to feel better makes you feel worse.

The cycle doesn't stop there. The guilt and shame you feel from emotional eating can become a new trigger, perpetuating the cycle. Feeling bad about overeating makes you more likely to seek comfort in food again. This creates a vicious loop that's difficult to break. The more you eat to cope with your emotions, the worse you feel, and the more you turn to food for relief. It's a self-reinforcing pattern that can leave you feeling trapped and hopeless.

Guilt and shame play are powerful emotions and can have a profound impact on your behavior. When you feel guilty about overeating, you might think, "I've already blown it; I might as well keep eating." This mindset can lead to further overeating and more guilt, creating a downward spiral. Self-criticism exacerbates the problem. Instead of offering yourself compassion and understanding, you berate yourself for not having more willpower. This negative self-talk can make you feel even more isolated and hopeless, driving you back to food for comfort.

The paradox of comfort eating is that it often leads to more distress. While the immediate act of eating can provide temporary relief, the long-term consequences are far from comforting. Emotional eating can lead to weight gain, health problems, and a strained relationship with food. These outcomes only add to your emotional burden, breaking the cycle even harder. It's a vicious loop that feeds on itself, making it increasingly difficult to find a way out.

Awareness is the first step in breaking this cycle. Recognizing that you're caught in this loop allows you to start making changes. You can start interrupting the cycle by becoming more aware of your emotional triggers and how you respond to them. When you feel the urge to eat emotionally, take a moment to pause and check in with yourself. Ask yourself what you feel and whether food is the best way to address those emotions.

Cognitive-behavioral techniques can also be effective. These techniques involve identifying and challenging the negative thoughts and beliefs contributing to emotional eating. For example, if you think, "I can't handle this stress without food," you can challenge that belief by reminding yourself of other coping strategies that have worked in the past. By changing your thought patterns, you can start to change your behavior.

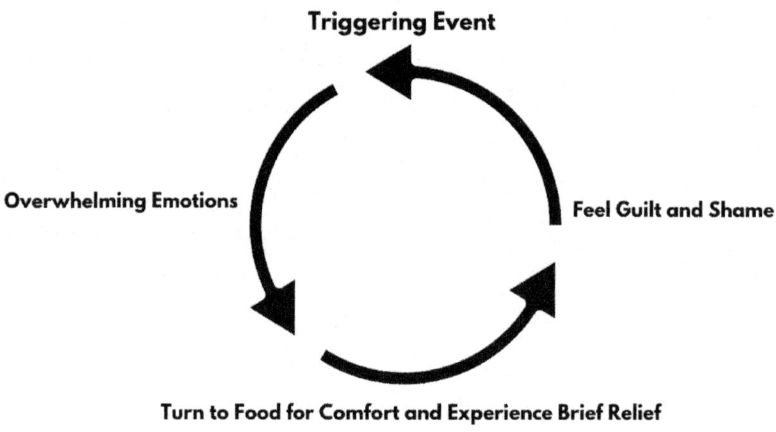

Several strategies can be used to disrupt the cycle of emotional eating. One approach is to identify alternative coping mechanisms. Instead of turning to food, find other ways to manage your emotions. This might involve talking to a friend, going for a walk, or engaging in a hobby you enjoy. The goal is to find activities that provide the same sense of comfort and distraction that food does but without the negative consequences.

Another important strategy is setting realistic, achievable goals. Instead of aiming to eliminate emotional eating overnight, set small, manageable goals that you can work towards gradually. For example, start by identifying one emotional eating trigger and finding a new way to cope. As you achieve these small goals, you'll build confidence, making tackling larger challenges easier.

Seeking professional help can also be beneficial. A therapist or counselor can provide valuable support and guidance as you work to break the cycle of emotional eating. They can help you explore the underlying emotions and experiences that contribute to your eating habits and develop strategies for managing them more effectively. If you struggle with specific mental health conditions like anxiety or depression, a mental health professional can also help you address these issues, reducing their impact on your eating behavior.

Recognizing the cycle of emotional eating and taking steps to disrupt it won't happen overnight. There will likely be setbacks along the way. But with awareness, self-compassion, and the right strategies, you can break free from the cycle and find better ways to manage your emotions.

THE IMPACT OF EMOTIONAL EATING ON MENTAL AND PHYSICAL HEALTH

Emotional eating doesn't just affect your waistline; it has profound implications for your mental health. When you use food to cope with emotions, it can lead to increased anxiety and depression. The temporary relief provided by eating is often followed by feelings of guilt and regret, which can exacerbate these mental health issues. It's a vicious cycle where food is used to numb emotional pain, but the aftermath of bingeing only adds to the emotional burden. Over time, this can create a pattern of emotional reliance

, to chronic feelings of anxiety and depression. You ...urself trapped in a cycle where the very act meant to ...becomes a source of distress.

...-esteem and body image issues are other significant ... health consequences of emotional eating. Frequently turning to food for comfort can lead to weight gain and body changes that may not align with societal beauty standards. This discrepancy can trigger a negative self-image and erode your self-esteem. You might find yourself avoiding social situations, feeling ashamed of your appearance, and constantly criticizing yourself. This negative self-talk further fuels emotional eating, creating a loop that's hard to break. It's important to recognize that your worth isn't tied to your body shape or size, but overcoming this mindset can be challenging when emotional eating is involved.

The sense of helplessness and lack of control accompanying emotional eating is also worth noting. When food becomes your primary coping mechanism, it can feel like you're at the mercy of your cravings and emotions. This lack of control can spill over into other areas of your life, making you feel powerless and overwhelmed. You might start to believe that you'll never break free from this cycle, which can diminish your motivation to seek healthier coping strategies. It's crucial to understand that while emotional eating may feel uncontrollable, there are steps you can take to regain your power and build a healthier relationship with food.

The impact of emotional eating can be just as severe to your physical health. One of the most immediate effects is weight gain and obesity. When you frequently consume high-calorie, high-fat foods in response to emotional triggers, your body stores the excess calories as fat. Over time, this can lead to significant weight gain and increase your risk of obesity. Furthermore, obesity itself is a risk factor for several chronic diseases, including diabetes and heart disease. The physical strain of carrying extra weight can also lead to joint pain, mobility issues, and a decreased quality of life.

Chronic diseases are another severe consequence of emotional eating. Consistently consuming sugary and fatty foods can lead to insulin resistance, a precursor to type 2 diabetes. High-fat diets can also result in elevated cholesterol levels, increasing the risk of heart disease. These health issues can become more complex when combined with the mental health challenges associated with emotional eating. For instance, the stress of managing a chronic disease can trigger more emotional eating, perpetuating a harmful cycle. It's important to recognize these risks and take proactive steps to address emotional eating before it leads to long-term health problems.

Digestive issues and poor nutrition are additional physical health concerns. Emotional eating often involves consuming large quantities of food quickly, which can overwhelm your digestive system. This can lead to symptoms like bloating, indigestion, and constipation. Moreover, the foods typically chosen for emotional eating are often low in nutrients and high in empty calories. Over time, this can result in nutrient deficiencies that affect your overall health and well-being. Poor nutrition can weaken your immune system, reduce energy levels, and impair your body's ability to function optimally. It's crucial to prioritize balanced nutrition to support your physical health and reduce the negative impacts of emotional eating.

Emotional, mental, and physical health interconnectedness cannot be overstated. Emotional eating affects all aspects of your well-being, creating a complex web of challenges that can be difficult to untangle. Addressing emotional eating requires a holistic approach, considering the interplay between your emotions, thoughts, and physical health. By focusing on holistic well-being, you can create a balanced and mindful approach to eating and self-care. This involves nurturing emotional health, practicing self-compassion, and prioritizing balanced nutrition and physical activity.

The benefits of a balanced, mindful approach to eating and self-care are profound. When you address emotional eating and prioritize holistic well-being, you can experience improved mental health, better physical health, and greater control and empowerment. This approach fosters a positive relationship with food and helps you develop healthier habits that support your overall well-being. It's not about perfection or eliminating emotional eating overnight; it's about making small, consistent changes that significantly improve your health and quality of life. By focusing on holistic well-being, you can break free from the cycle of emotional eating and build a healthier, more balanced future.

CHAPTER 2

IDENTIFYING AND MANAGING TRIGGERS

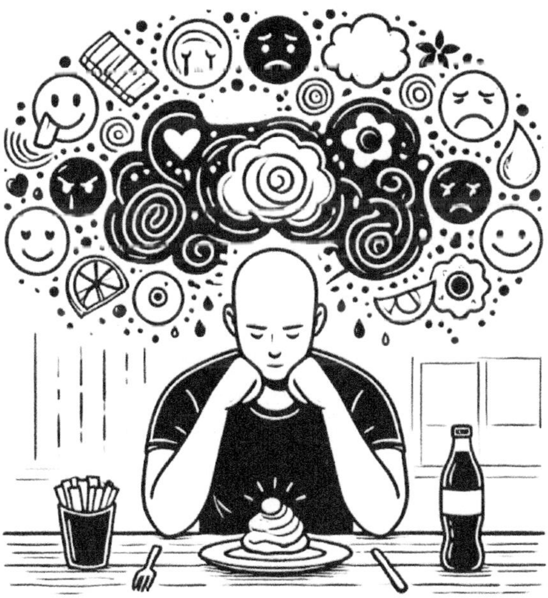

Am sure you are familiar with this scenario. You are at your desk at work as emails keep flooding in. Your boss just assigned an urgent task, and your stress levels are skyrocketing. Without thinking, you reach for that stash of candy in your drawer. Before you know it, it is all gone. You weren't hungry, but eating offered a momentary escape from the stress. This is a common scenario for many people who struggle with emotional eating. The key to overcoming this habit is understanding and managing your triggers.

EMOTIONAL TRIGGERS: STRESS, SADNESS, AND BEYOND

Different emotions can push you toward emotional eating. Stress is one of the most common triggers. When stressed, your body releases cortisol, increasing your appetite, particularly for high-fat, sugary foods, as previously discussed. These foods provide a quick energy boost, but the relief is temporary. Once the cortisol levels drop, the cravings subside, but the cycle often repeats, trapping you in a loop of stress and eating.

Sadness and loneliness are also other powerful triggers. Food can become a source of comfort when you're feeling down or isolated. Imagine coming home to an empty house after a long day. The silence feels heavy, and you reach for any sweet food in the pantry. The sweetness provides a fleeting sense of comfort, temporarily lifting your spirits but often leaving you feeling worse afterward. It's a cycle that can be hard to break.

Interestingly, even positive emotions like happiness can trigger emotional eating. Celebrations often revolve around food, whether it's a birthday, a promotion, or a holiday. These events can lead to overeating, not because you're hungry, but because food is tied to the joy and excitement of the occasion. Think about the last time you went to a party. You might have been eating more than usual simply because the atmosphere was festive, and the food was plentiful.

To manage these emotional triggers, you need effective strategies for emotional regulation. Deep breathing exercises can be a simple yet powerful tool. When you feel a craving coming on, take a few deep breaths. Close your eyes, inhale deeply through your nose, hold for a few seconds, and then exhale slowly through your mouth. This helps calm your nervous system and gives you a moment to think before you reach for food.

Progressive muscle relaxation is another technique that can help. This involves tensing and slowly releasing different muscle groups from your head to your toes. This method helps reduce physical tension and shifts your focus away from the craving and onto your body, helping you become more aware of your physical state.

Mindfulness meditation can also be incredibly effective. Take a few minutes daily to sit quietly and focus on your breath. Notice your thoughts and feelings without judgment. If you feel a craving, acknowledge it, but don't act on it immediately. Instead, try to understand what emotion is driving the craving. Are you stressed? Lonely? Happy? By identifying the root emotion, you can address it directly rather than using food as a temporary fix.

Incorporating these techniques into your daily routine can help you build resilience against emotional triggers. Create a toolkit of strategies when emotions threaten to overwhelm you. The more you practice, the easier it becomes to recognize your triggers and choose healthier coping methods.

ENVIRONMENTAL TRIGGERS: HOW YOUR SURROUNDINGS INFLUENCE EATING

Different environments can also prompt emotional eating, and the presence of easily accessible junk food is a common culprit. When snacks are within arm's reach, resisting the temptation is much more complicated, especially when feeling vulnerable or stressed.

Eating out in social settings can also trigger emotional eating. Imagine going to a restaurant with friends. The atmosphere is lively, and everyone orders appetizers, entrees, and desserts. Getting caught up in the moment and overeating is easy, even if you aren't starving. Social settings often come with pressures and expectations, making it challenging to stick to mindful eating habits.

Daily routines and habits play a significant role in emotional eating. Evening routines can lead to snacking. After dinner, you might find yourself settling down to watch TV. Watching TV becomes associated with snacking; before you know it, you're reaching for a bowl of popcorn. It's not about hunger; it's about habit. Associating certain activities with eating can create a vital link in your mind, making it difficult to break the cycle.

It's crucial to create a supportive environment to manage these environmental triggers. One practical tip is to keep healthy snacks available. Stock your fridge and pantry with nutritious options like fruits, vegetables, nuts, and yogurt. When healthy choices are readily accessible, you're more likely to reach for them instead of junk food.

Redesigning your kitchen and pantry can make a big difference. Place healthier items at eye level and store less healthy options out of sight or in hard-to-reach places. You can reduce the temptation to indulge in emotional eating by making minor environmental adjustments.

Setting boundaries for eating at specific times and places can help, too. Designate certain areas of your home for eating, such as the dining table, and avoid eating in front of the TV or your bedroom. This creates a clear separation between activities and helps you become more mindful of when and where you eat. Setting a schedule for meals and snacks can also prevent mindless eating. By planning your eating times, you can ensure that you're eating because you're hungry, not because you're bored or stressed.

PSYCHOLOGICAL TRIGGERS: UNDERSTANDING YOUR MIND'S ROLE

You might not realize it, but your thoughts can significantly impact your eating habits. Cognitive distortions, or distorted thinking patterns, often play a significant role in emotional eating. One common cognitive distortion is all-or-nothing thinking. This is when you view things in black-and-white terms. For example, you might think, "I've already eaten one cookie, so I might as well eat the whole bag." This kind of thinking doesn't allow for moderation and can lead to bingeing. Instead of enjoying a treat and moving on, you are spiraling into overeating because you feel like you've already "failed."

Another cognitive distortion is catastrophizing. This is when you blow things out of proportion. You might eat a slice of cake and then think, "I've completely ruined my diet, and now I'll never lose weight." This extreme thinking can trigger feelings of guilt and shame, which can lead to more emotional eating. Recognizing these distorted thought patterns is the first step in managing them. It's important to understand that one slip-up doesn't ruin all your efforts. Every meal is a new opportunity to make a healthier choice.

Negative self-talk is another psychological trigger that can lead to emotional eating. The way you talk to yourself matters. Constantly criticizing yourself can erode your self-esteem and make you more likely to turn to food for comfort. Identifying these negative thoughts can be challenging. You might find yourself thinking, "I'm so fat," or "I'll never be able to control my eating." These thoughts can become a self-fulfilling prophecy if left unchecked.

Transforming negative self-talk into positive affirmations can make a big difference. Instead of saying, "I'm so fat," try saying, "I'm working on becoming healthier every day." Instead of, "I'll never be able to control my eating," say, "I'm learning new ways to manage my emotions without food." Positive affirmations can help shift your mindset and build your self-esteem. They remind you that change is possible and that you have the power to make healthier choices.

Cognitive-behavioral techniques can also be very effective in managing psychological triggers. Thought challenging and reframing are two such techniques. Thought challenging involves questioning the validity of your negative thoughts. Ask yourself, "Is this thought based on fact or emotion?" "What evidence do I have to support this thought?" By challenging your negative thoughts, you can see them in a new light. Reframing involves changing the way you think about a situation. Instead of viewing a mistake as a failure, see it as a learning opportunity. This shift in perspective can reduce the emotional impact of your thoughts and make it easier to manage your eating habits.

Behavioral experiments are another cognitive-behavioral technique that can help. These involve testing new behaviors to see how they affect your thoughts and feelings. For example, if you tend to eat when bored, try finding a different activity, like walking or reading a book. Notice how this new behavior affects your mood and your desire to eat. By experimenting with other behaviors, you can find new ways to manage your emotions without turning to food.

Expert insights can provide valuable guidance on managing psychological triggers. Cognitive-behavioral therapists often emphasize the importance of being aware of your thoughts and how they influence your behavior. Dr. Aaron Beck, a pioneer in cognitive-behavioral therapy, states, "Our thoughts are the lens through which we view the world. By changing our thoughts, we can change our world experience." Research has shown that cognitive-behavioral techniques can effectively manage emotional eating. A study published in the journal "Appetite" found that individuals who used cognitive-behavioral strategies significantly reduced emotional eating compared to those who did not.

JOURNALING AND SELF-REFLECTION

Journaling can be a powerful tool for identifying and managing emotional eating triggers. When you take the time to write down your thoughts and feelings, you create a space for reflection and self-awareness. This practice helps you track your emotions and eating habits, making it easier to spot patterns and triggers. Journaling allows you to step back and see the bigger picture rather than getting lost in the daily hustle and bustle. By documenting your experiences, you can gain insights into what drives your emotional eating and develop strategies to address it.

One of the key benefits of journaling is that it helps you track your emotions alongside your eating habits. For instance, you might notice that you tend to reach for snacks when feeling anxious or bored. By writing down these observations, you can understand the emotional cues leading to eating. Reflective journaling takes this further by encouraging you to explore the deeper reasons behind your actions. You might ask yourself why certain emotions trigger the need to eat and what alternative ways you could manage those feelings.

To get you started, here are some specific journaling prompts designed to help you explore your triggers. One prompt could be, "What emotions did I feel before I ate?" This question encourages you to think about the emotional state you were in before you reached for food. Were you stressed, sad, or perhaps even happy? Another useful prompt is, "What was happening around me when I decided to eat?" This helps you consider the environmental factors that might have influenced your decision. Were you alone or with others? Were you watching TV or scrolling through your phone?

As you engage in these journaling exercises, you'll see patterns emerge. You might realize that you often eat when you're lonely or that certain situations, like watching TV, trigger mindless snacking. By identifying these patterns, you can start to develop strategies to manage them. For example, if you notice that you eat out of boredom, you could plan engaging activities to keep yourself occupied during those times. If stress is a trigger, you might explore relaxation techniques to help you unwind without turning to food.

Self-reflection plays a crucial role in this process. Reflecting on your past eating episodes allows you to better understand your behaviors and motivations. It's about more than just noting what you ate but why. Reflecting on these moments can help you identify alternative actions to take in the future. For instance, instead of reaching for a snack when you're stressed, you might go for a walk, practice deep breathing, or call a friend. These alternative actions can provide the emotional relief you need without turning to food.

Journaling Prompts

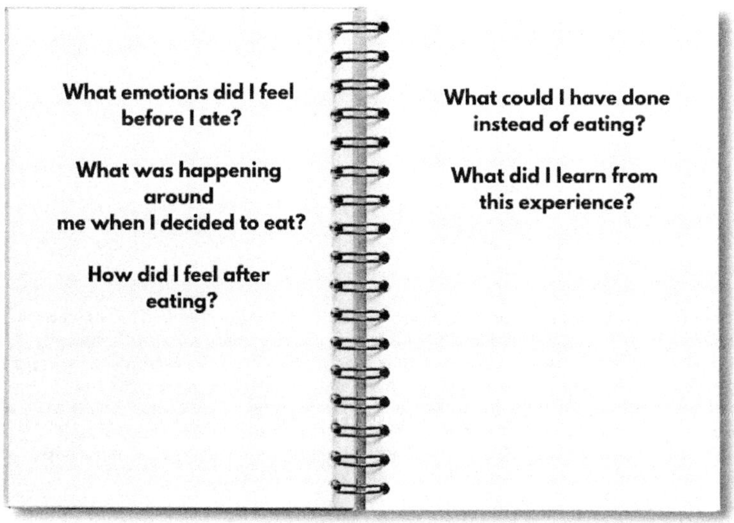

Use these prompts to guide your journaling practice. Set aside a few minutes daily to reflect on your eating habits and emotions. Over time, you'll build a clearer picture of your triggers and develop healthier ways to manage them. The key is to approach this practice with curiosity and self-compassion. Remember, the goal is not to judge yourself but to understand and support yourself better.

As you continue to journal and reflect, your awareness and control over your eating habits will improve. You'll start to recognize the emotional cues that lead to eating and feel more empowered to choose alternative ways to cope. This process takes time and patience, but the insights you gain can be invaluable in your journey. By making journaling and self-reflection a regular part of your routine, you can cultivate a deeper understanding of yourself and your triggers, paving the way for lasting change.

Stories of Identifying Triggers

Let's explore real-life examples to illustrate how people identify and manage emotional eating triggers.

Emily's Story

Meet Emily, a college student who struggled with stress-related eating. Finals week was always her worst time. She'd find herself surrounded by empty takeout containers, chips, and candy wrappers as she crammed for exams. The stress of academic pressure pushed her to seek comfort in food, and this habit was affecting her health and academic performance. It wasn't until she started keeping a food diary that she noticed a pattern. Emily tracked not just what she ate but also how she felt each time she reached for a snack. She realized that her bingeing episodes always coincided with high-stress periods. This awareness was her first step toward change.

Emily sought help from her university's counseling center, where she joined a support group for students dealing with stress and anxiety. Through group discussions, she learned she wasn't alone in her struggles. The camaraderie and shared experiences provided her with emotional support and practical advice. She started practicing mindfulness exercises to manage her stress. She found healthier coping methods, like taking short walks or practicing deep breathing techniques. Emily faced challenges along the way, especially the initial resistance to change. It was easier to reach for junk food than to confront her stress head-on. But with consistency and discipline, she gradually overcame these obstacles.

Mark's Story

Mark, a busy working parent, often snacked late at night after putting the kids to bed. It became a routine: a beer, a bag of chips, and a couple of hours in front of the TV. He knew it wasn't healthy, but it felt like his only way to unwind after a long day. Mark decided to take a closer look at his habits. He started by keeping a food diary and noticed that his snacking was tied to specific activities, like watching TV. This realization prompted him to make changes to his environment.

Mark reorganized his kitchen and pantry, moving unhealthy snacks to higher shelves and placing fruits and vegetables within easy reach. He also set boundaries for eating, deciding that the living room was off-limits for food. Instead, he designated the dining table as the only place for meals and snacks. This small change made a big difference. Mark also involved his family in his efforts, creating a supportive home environment where everyone was encouraged to make healthier choices. The process had its challenges. There were nights when he found it hard to resist the lure of the couch and a bag of chips. But over time, he developed new routines that didn't revolve around food.

Both Emily and Mark faced significant challenges in their journeys. Emily struggled with consistency, often reverting to old habits during particularly stressful times. Mark found it difficult to break the association between certain activities and eating. Yet, both persevered, using the insights they gained from tracking their patterns and seeking support. Their efforts led to positive outcomes. Emily noticed a significant improvement in her mental health and academic performance. She felt more in control of her eating habits and experienced fewer binge episodes. Mark found that his new routines helped him manage his weight and improved his overall well-being. He felt more energetic and less reliant on food for emotional comfort.

Their experiences show that while the journey may be challenging, the outcomes are worth the effort. Attainable goals are improved mental health, better physical well-being, and a healthier relationship with food. As you reflect on these examples, consider how you can apply similar strategies to your own life. Remember, the first step is awareness. Start by tracking your patterns, seek support, and be patient with yourself.

Recognizing and addressing triggers forms the cornerstone of conquering emotional eating. By gaining insight into the motivations behind your eating habits, you can create effective methods to counteract them.

CHAPTER 3

CULTIVATING MINDFUL EATING PRACTICES

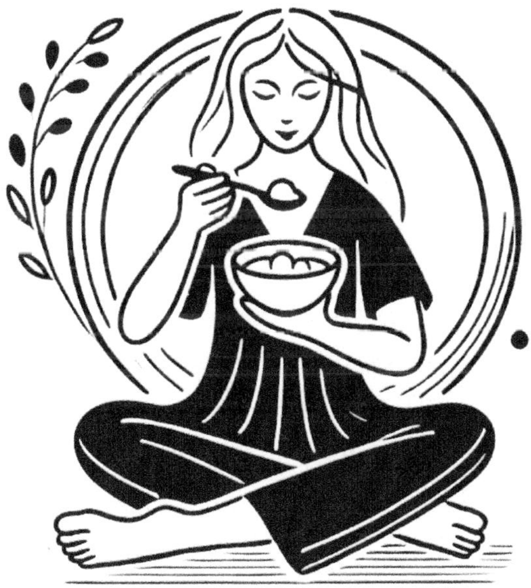

One evening, after a particularly stressful day, I stood in the kitchen, mindlessly eating a box of crackers. Before I knew it, the box was empty, and I couldn't even remember tasting the crackers! This was a wake-up call for me. I realized that I needed to change how I approached eating and how I related to food. This is where mindful eating comes into play.

WHAT IS MINDFUL EATING?

Mindful eating is about being fully present during meals. It involves paying attention to the eating experience, from the flavors and textures of the food to the sensations of hunger and fullness in your body. Unlike mindless eating, where you might eat on autopilot, mindful eating encourages you to slow down and savor each bite. It's about appreciating your food and the act of eating without distraction. When you eat mindfully, you tune into your body's signals, recognizing when you're hungry and satisfied, which can help you make healthier choices.

One of the critical aspects of mindful eating is awareness of physical hunger and satiety cues. Before you eat, take a moment to check in with your body. Are you eating because you're physically hungry, or are you eating to fill an emotional void? By distinguishing between these two types of hunger, you can make more informed decisions about when and what to eat. As you eat, pay attention to how your body feels. Notice when you start feeling full and satisfied and allow yourself to stop eating. This can help prevent overeating and promote a healthier relationship with food.

The benefits of mindful eating extend beyond just reducing binge-eating episodes. When you eat mindfully, you give your body the time it needs to properly digest food, improving digestion and leading to greater satisfaction with meals. Instead of feeling bloated or uncomfortable after eating, you'll feel more in tune with your body's needs. Mindful eating can also enhance your mental well-being by reducing stress and anxiety around food. When you approach eating with mindfulness, you create a sense of calm and presence that can carry over into other areas of your life.

Mindful eating stands in stark contrast to mindless eating. Mindless eating often occurs when you're distracted, such as in front of the TV or while scrolling through your phone. In these situations, you're not paying attention to the food or your body's signals, which can lead to overeating and a lack of satisfaction. Rushing through meals is another form of mindless eating. When you eat quickly, you don't give your body enough time to register fullness, and you miss out on enjoying the meal. In contrast, mindful eating encourages you to slow down, savor each bite, and fully engage with the eating experience.

The principles of mindfulness can be applied to eating in several ways. One of the core principles is non-judgmental awareness. This means observing your thoughts, feelings, and sensations without judging them as good or bad. When you eat mindfully, you pay attention to your body's signals and the sensory experience of eating without criticism or judgment. If you eat when you're not hungry or eating more than you intended, acknowledge it without guilt or shame. This non-judgmental approach allows you to learn from your experiences and make healthier choices in the future.

Another essential principle is acceptance of the current experience. This means being present with whatever is happening, whether it's a craving, a feeling of fullness, or an emotional trigger.

By accepting your experience without trying to change or push it away, you can respond to your body's needs with greater compassion and understanding. For example, if you notice a craving for a specific food, instead of immediately acting on it, take a moment to explore what might be driving that craving. Are you feeling stressed, bored, or lonely? By accepting and examining your current experience, you can address the underlying emotion and make a more mindful choice.

Mindfullness Exercise

- ☐ Take a small piece of food, such as a raisin or chocolate.
- ☐ Hold it in your hand and observe it closely. Notice its color, texture, and shape.
- ☐ Bring the food to your nose and take a moment to smell it. Notice the aroma and any sensations it evokes.
- ☐ Place the food in your mouth, but don't immediately chew it. Notice how it feels on your tongue.
- ☐ Slowly begin to chew, paying attention to the flavors and textures. Chew thoroughly and savor each bite.
- ☐ As you swallow, notice how your body feels. Are you more aware of your hunger and fullness signals?

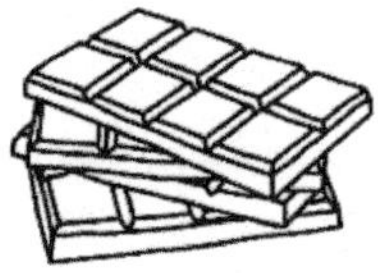

This exercise can help you practice mindful eating and increase awareness of your eating habits.

STRATEGIES FOR PRACTICING MINDFULNESS AT MEALTIMES

Creating a mindful eating environment is one of the first steps to changing your relationship with food. Eating in a quiet, distraction-free space can make a significant difference. Turn off the TV, put your phone away, and choose a spot to sit comfortably. This might be your dining table, a cozy kitchen corner, or even a quiet place outside. By dedicating a specific space for eating, you signal to your mind that this time is for nourishment and presence.

Using appealing table settings and utensils can also enhance your mindful eating experience. Use your favorite plates, bowls, and utensils. Maybe light a candle or arrange some flowers on the table. These small touches can transform a simple meal into a more meaningful experience. When your surroundings are pleasant, you're more likely to slow down and appreciate each bite.

Before taking your first bite, consider introducing pre-meal rituals to center yourself. Taking a few deep breaths can help you shift from a state of stress or distraction to one of calm and focus. Sit comfortably, close your eyes, and take a few deep breaths. Inhale deeply through your nose, hold for a moment, and then exhale slowly through your mouth. Repeat this a few times until you feel more centered. Another powerful pre-meal ritual is expressing gratitude for your food. Take a moment to acknowledge your food's journey to reach your plate, from those who grew it to the hands that prepared it. This simple gratitude can create a deeper connection with your meal and set a positive tone for your eating experience.

Once you're ready to eat, the goal should be to remain present and fully engaged with your meal. Start by chewing slowly and thoroughly. Take smaller bites and chew each one several times before swallowing. This not only aids digestion but also allows you to savor the flavors and textures of your food. Pausing between bites to assess your hunger levels can also be beneficial. Put your fork down between bites and take a moment to check in with yourself. Are you still hungry, or are you starting to feel full? This pause gives your body time to signal satiety, helping you avoid overeating.

Noticing your food's flavors, textures, and aromas is another crucial aspect of mindful eating. As you chew, pay attention to the different tastes and sensations in your mouth. Is the food sweet, salty, sour, or bitter? Is it crunchy, smooth, or creamy? Engaging your senses can make the eating experience more enjoyable and satisfying. It also helps you stay present and focused on eating rather than letting your mind wander.

Guided mindfulness exercises can further enhance your mindful eating practice. A five-minute pre-meal meditation can set the stage for a mindful meal. Find a comfortable seat, close your eyes, and take a few deep breaths. Focus on your breath, noticing the sensation of the air entering and leaving your nostrils. If your mind wanders, gently bring your focus back to your breath. After a few minutes, shift your attention to your body, noticing any sensations of hunger or fullness. This simple meditation can help you tune into your body's signals and create a sense of calm before eating.

A guided body scan focusing on hunger cues can also be helpful. Sit comfortably and close your eyes. Starting at the top of your head, slowly scan down through your body, noticing any sensations of hunger or fullness. Pay attention to your stomach, seeing if it feels empty, full, or somewhere in between. This body scan can help you become more aware of your physical hunger cues, making distinguishing between true hunger and emotional cravings easier.

Creating a supportive environment, introducing pre-meal rituals, practicing mindful eating techniques, and using guided mindfulness exercises can all help you stay present and engaged with your food. This not only enhances your eating experience but also supports your overall well-being.

RECOGNIZING PHYSICAL HUNGER VERSUS EMOTIONAL HUNGER

As previously discussed, one of the biggest challenges in overcoming emotional eating is distinguishing between physical and emotional hunger. Physical hunger is your body's natural signal that it needs nourishment. It builds gradually, starting with subtle cues like a slight emptiness in your stomach. It intensifies over time if not addressed. Physical hunger can usually be satisfied with various foods, whether a hearty salad, a bowl of soup, or a sandwich. You know you're physically hungry when you experience cues like stomach growling, low energy levels, or physical discomfort from prolonged hunger. These signals are your body's way of telling you it needs fuel to function properly.

On the other hand, emotional hunger is driven by emotional needs rather than physical ones. It often comes on suddenly and feels urgent. You might crave comfort foods like chocolate, chips, or ice cream. These cravings are usually tied to your emotional state rather than your body's need for nutrients. Unlike physical hunger, emotional hunger can lead to guilt or shame after eating, as you realize you weren't starving in the first place.

To help you differentiate between physical and emotional hunger, consider using practical tools like the hunger and fullness scale. This scale ranges from 1 to 10, with 1 being extremely hungry and 10 being uncomfortably full. Before you eat, take a moment to rate your hunger on this scale. If you're at a 3 or 4, you're likely experiencing physical hunger and can benefit from eating. If you're at a 7 or 8, you might be eating out of habit or emotional need rather than actual hunger. This simple tool can help you become more aware of your hunger cues and make more mindful eating choices.

SAVORING EACH BITE: TECHNIQUES FOR ENGAGING YOUR SENSES

Imagine sitting down to a meal where every bite is a new experience, where you fully engage with the food on your plate. This is the essence of sensory engagement, a practice that can transform how you eat. By using all your senses—sight, smell, taste, touch, and even sound—you can deepen your connection with your food and enhance your eating experience.

To start, consider the visual appeal of your meal. Before taking your first bite, take a moment to observe the colors and presentation of the food. Notice the vibrant greens of the vegetables, the rich browns of the roasted meat, or the bright reds of a fresh tomato. The visual aspect can set the stage for the entire meal, making it more inviting and enjoyable. When food looks appealing, you're more likely to appreciate and savor it.

Next, take a deep breath and bring the food closer to your nose. Smelling the aroma of your meal can trigger your digestive juices and prepare your body for eating. The scent of freshly baked bread, the tang of citrus, or the earthy aroma of roasted vegetables can evoke a sense of anticipation and pleasure. Smelling your food before eating can also help you slow down and become more present in the moment.

As you take your first bite, focus on the texture and flavor. Notice how the food feels in your mouth. Is it crunchy, smooth, or chewy? Pay attention to the different flavors that unfold as you chew. Is it sweet, salty, bitter, or umami? Chewing slowly and thoroughly allows you to fully experience these sensations. Each bite becomes an opportunity to explore and enjoy the complexities of your meal.

Touch plays a role in sensory engagement, too. Feel the weight of your fork or spoon, the texture of the napkin, or the coolness of a glass of water. These tactile sensations contribute to the overall dining experience. You can create a more immersive eating environment by engaging your sense of touch.

Even sound can enhance your meal. The crunch of a fresh apple, the sizzle of a hot skillet, or the gentle clinking of cutlery can add another layer of sensory enjoyment. These sounds can ground you in the present moment, making each bite more meaningful.

Savoring each bite has several benefits. It can lead to increased meal enjoyment as you become more attuned to the flavors and textures of your food. This heightened awareness can make meals more satisfying, reducing the urge to overeat. Savoring also promotes better digestion and nutrient absorption. When you chew thoroughly and eat slowly, your digestive system has more time to process the food, improving digestion and overall health.

Another practical exercise is guided tasting. Select a variety of foods with different textures and flavors. Take small bites and focus on one aspect at a time. Notice the crunchiness of a carrot, an avocado's creaminess, or a berry's sweetness. Focusing on these details can enhance sensory engagement and make each meal more enjoyable.

By using sight, smell, taste, touch, and sound, you can fully experience and appreciate each meal. This practice can lead to greater satisfaction, improved digestion, and a deeper connection with your food.

OVERCOMING MINDLESS EATING: TOOLS FOR STAYING PRESENT

Many of us fall into mindless eating habits without even realizing it. Speed eating is another common culprit. In our fast-paced world, it's tempting to rush through meals, barely chewing and not truly tasting your food. This can lead to overeating because you don't give your body enough time to register fullness.

To stay present during meals, start by setting aside dedicated mealtimes. This means carving out specific times in your day solely for eating. Treat these times as sacred, uninterrupted moments. Removing distractions is very important. Turn off the TV, silence your phone, and close your laptop. The goal should be to focus entirely on the act of eating. This helps you become more aware of what you're eating and how much, making it easier to recognize when you're full.

Pay attention to each bite of food. Chew slowly and thoroughly. Notice how the food feels in your mouth. This mindful approach enhances your eating experience and helps you detect satiety signals, preventing overeating. Being present gives your body the time it needs to communicate that it's had enough.

When you stay present, you become more attuned to your body's cues. Recognizing fullness signals is a key aspect of this. As you eat, periodically check in with yourself. Are you still hungry, or are you starting to feel satisfied? This awareness helps you stop eating when you're full rather than mindlessly continuing until you're uncomfortable. Eating slower is another effective strategy. When you slow down, you give your body time to process the food and signal your brain that you're full. This can help you avoid the discomfort and guilt that often accompany overeating.

As we wrap up this chapter, remember that mindful eating is a powerful tool for overcoming emotional eating. You can develop a more balanced relationship with food by staying present and engaged with your meals.

CHAPTER 4

BUILDING A TOOLBOX OF COPING STRATEGIES

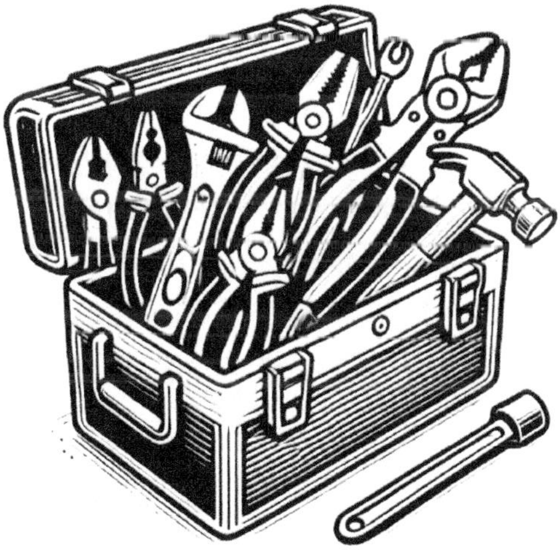

You're stuck in traffic after a long day at work. The frustration builds with every minute, and by the time you get home, all you can think about is diving into the jar of sweets on the kitchen counter. This scenario might sound all too familiar. When stress or emotions run high, seeking comfort in food is common. But what if you had other tools at your disposal to cope with these feelings? This chapter is about building a toolbox with strategies to help you manage your emotions without turning to food.

THOUGHT RECORDS

One practical exercise to manage your emotions is keeping thought records. Start by tracking your negative thoughts and analyzing them. Write down the situation that triggered the thought, the thought itself, and the emotion it elicited. Then, challenge the thought by asking questions like, "Is this thought based on fact or emotion?" and "What evidence do I have to support or refute this thought?" Reframe the thought into a more balanced or neutral statement. For example, if you think, "I'll never be able to control my eating," reframe it to, "I'm learning new ways to manage my emotions without food, and I can make progress over time."

Behavioral activation is another technique that can help increase positive activities in your life. When you're feeling down or stressed, it's easy to withdraw and avoid activities you once enjoyed. Behavioral activation encourages you to engage in activities that bring you joy and fulfillment. Start by making a list of activities you have enjoyed or have enjoyed. These could be anything from walking in nature to painting or playing a musical instrument. Schedule time for these activities in your week, even if you don't feel like doing them at first. Positive activities can lift your mood and provide healthier ways to cope with emotions.

STRESS MANAGEMENT: YOGA, MEDITATION, AND BREATHING EXERCISES

Managing stress is crucial for overcoming emotional eating. Effective stress management can lower cortisol levels, reduce cravings, and improve emotional resilience. Yoga, meditation, and breathing exercises are powerful tools for managing stress and promoting a sense of calm and balance.

Yoga is an excellent practice for stress relief, offering a combination of physical movement and mental relaxation. Specific yoga poses can help alleviate stress and calm your nervous system.

- Child's pose, for example, is a simple yet effective pose for relaxation. To do this pose, kneel on the floor, sit back on your heels, and stretch your arms forward while resting your forehead on the mat. This pose stretches your back and shoulders, promoting a sense of calm and relaxation.
- Legs-up-the-wall pose is another great option for calming the nervous system. Lie on your back with your legs extended up against a wall, creating a gentle inversion that helps reduce stress and improve circulation.
- Sun salutations, a series of flowing movements, can help reduce stress by combining breath and movement, promoting balance and well-being.

Meditation is another powerful tool for managing stress. Guided meditation practices can help you cultivate mindfulness and reduce anxiety. Body scan meditation is a technique where you mentally scan your body from head to toe, noticing any areas of tension or discomfort. This practice helps you become more aware of your physical sensations and promotes relaxation. Loving-kindness meditation, or "metta" meditation, involves silently repeating phrases that send love and compassion to yourself and others. For example, you might say, "May I be happy, may I be healthy, may I be safe." This practice can help you develop a more compassionate and positive mindset, reducing stress and promoting emotional well-being.

Breathing exercises are another effective way to manage stress. Diaphragmatic breathing, or "belly breathing," involves taking deep breaths that fully engage your diaphragm. To practice this, sit or lie comfortably and place one hand on your chest and the other on your belly. Take a deep breath through your nose, then exhale slowly through your mouth. This type of breathing helps activate the body's relaxation response, reducing stress and promoting calm. The 4-7-8 breathing technique is another helpful exercise. Inhale deeply through your nose for a count of four, hold your breath for a count of seven, and then exhale slowly through your mouth for a count of eight. This technique can help calm your nervous system and reduce anxiety. Alternate nostril breathing is breathing through one nostril at a time while closing the other with your fingers. This exercise helps balance your brain's left and right hemispheres, promoting a sense of calm and balance.

These stress management techniques can be powerful tools. Incorporating yoga, meditation, and breathing exercises into your daily routine can reduce cortisol levels, improve emotional resilience, and develop healthier coping methods. Remember, it's not about eliminating stress entirely but finding effective ways to manage it and reduce its impact on your eating habits.

CREATIVE OUTLETS: ART, WRITING, AND MUSIC AS THERAPY

Engaging in creative activities can be a powerful way to manage emotions, offering a form of expression that words alone often can't capture. Art, writing, and music provide therapeutic benefits by allowing you to externalize your feelings, offering a sense of catharsis.

Art offers a unique way to express feelings that might be difficult to articulate. You don't need to be a skilled artist to benefit from this form of therapy. The act of creating itself is what's important. Mandala coloring, for instance, is a simple yet effective activity that promotes relaxation. The repetitive patterns and focus required to color within the lines can help calm your mind, providing a meditative experience. Free-form painting is another excellent option. Here, you allow your emotions to guide your brush without worrying about creating a "perfect" piece. This freedom can help release pent-up emotions and offer a sense of relief. The colors and shapes you choose can reflect your inner state, turning abstract feelings into something tangible.

Writing is another powerful outlet for managing emotions. Journaling allows you to explore and understand your feelings, providing a space to be completely honest. Stream-of-consciousness writing, where you write continuously without worrying about grammar or structure, can help you tap into your subconscious mind, revealing thoughts and emotions you might not have been aware of. Writing letters to yourself is another therapeutic exercise. You can write a letter to your past self, offering forgiveness and understanding, or to your future self, expressing hopes and goals. Poetry and storytelling can also be emotional outlets, allowing you to explore your feelings through creative narratives.

The act of writing can help you process emotions and gain new perspectives.

Music therapy offers another dimension of emotional regulation. Music profoundly affects mood and can be used to manage various emotional states. Creating personal playlists tailored to different moods can be a practical tool. For instance, you might have a relaxing playlist filled with calming instrumental tracks and another for motivation, featuring upbeat songs that boost your energy. Playing musical instruments is another form of expression. Whether strumming a guitar, playing the piano, or drumming, the physical act of making music can provide an emotional release. The vibrations and rhythms can resonate with your inner state, helping you process emotions through sound.

Create A Personal Playlist!

Create a playlist for relaxation: Choose songs that calm your mind and help you unwind.

Create a playlist for motivation: Select upbeat, energizing tracks that lift your spirits.

Create a playlist for reflection: Include songs encouraging introspection and emotional exploration.

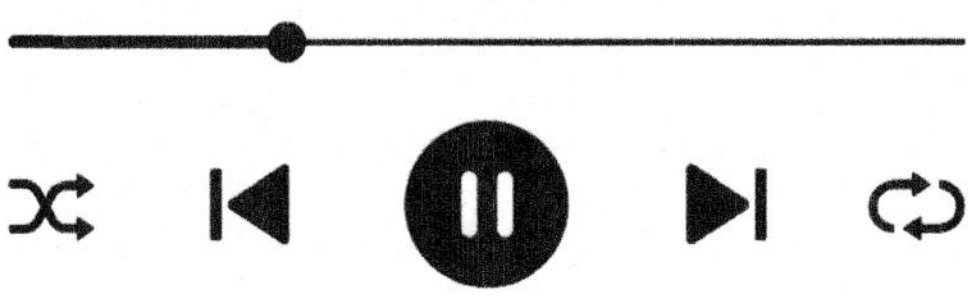

These creative outlets—art, writing, and music—offer different ways to explore and express emotions. They can help you manage stress, process feelings, and find a sense of balance. Engaging in these activities regularly can build emotional resilience and provide healthy ways to cope with life's challenges.

PHYSICAL ACTIVITY: EXERCISE AS A MOOD ENHANCER

Exercise has a profound impact on your mood. When you engage in physical activity, your body releases endorphins, also known as "feel-good" hormones. These chemicals interact with receptors in your brain to reduce pain perception and trigger a positive feeling in the body. This natural high can lift your spirits and provide a healthy coping mechanism for stress and anxiety.

Another significant benefit of exercise is the reduction of stress hormones like cortisol. Incorporating regular physical activity into your routine can help keep cortisol levels in check, reducing cravings. Exercise also promotes better sleep, which further helps to regulate stress hormones and improve overall mood. You're better equipped to handle emotional triggers without turning to food when well-rested.

There are many exercises to choose from, catering to different preferences and fitness levels. Cardiovascular exercises like running and swimming considerably increase heart rate and boost endorphin levels. These activities can be done solo or in groups, making them versatile options. Strength training, including weightlifting and resistance band exercises, helps build muscle and improve overall strength. It also has the added benefit of increasing your metabolism and aiding in weight management. For those who prefer a more relaxed approach, recreational activities like dancing, hiking, or playing sports can provide physical and emotional benefits. These activities are enjoyable and offer a sense of accomplishment and community.

Consistency is key when it comes to reaping the benefits of physical activity. Creating a weekly exercise routine can help you stay on track and make exercise a regular part of your life. Start by setting realistic fitness goals that align with your current abilities and gradually increase the intensity and duration of your workouts. This approach helps prevent burnout and reduces the risk of injury. For example, if you're new to exercise, begin with short, manageable sessions like a 20-minute walk three times a week. As you build endurance, you can gradually increase the duration and frequency of your workouts.

Staying motivated to exercise can be challenging, but there are several strategies to keep you on track. Finding a workout buddy can make exercising more enjoyable and provide accountability. You can encourage each other, share progress, and even try new activities together. Joining community fitness groups or classes can also provide a sense of belonging and support. Whether it's a local running club, a dance class, or a group fitness session at the gym, being part of a community can make exercise more fun and less of a chore.

Tracking your progress with fitness apps can be another effective way to stay motivated. Many apps allow you to set goals, log workouts, and monitor your progress over time. Seeing your improvements can boost your confidence and keep you motivated to continue. Some apps even offer virtual challenges and rewards, adding excitement to your fitness journey. Additionally, consider rewarding yourself for reaching milestones. Treat yourself to something special, like a new workout outfit or a relaxing massage, to celebrate your achievements.

Incorporating physical activity into your daily routine enhances your mood and provides a healthy outlet for managing emotions. You can make exercise a rewarding part of your life by choosing activities you enjoy, staying consistent, and using motivational strategies.

BUILDING A SUPPORT NETWORK: FRIENDS, FAMILY, AND PROFESSIONAL HELP

When you're struggling with emotional eating, having a strong support network can make a world of difference. Trying to overcome your challenges alone without anyone to lean on is overwhelming! A support network offers emotional encouragement, understanding, and accountability. It's like having a safety net that catches you when you stumble. Friends and family who understand your struggles can offer a shoulder to cry on, a listening ear, or even a gentle nudge when needed. They can be your cheerleaders, celebrating successes and helping you navigate setbacks.

But how do you build this support network? Start by reaching out to those closest to you. Share your struggles and goals with friends and family. Be open and honest about what you're going through and what kind of support you need. You might be surprised at how willing people are to help when they understand what you're facing. Sometimes, having someone to talk to makes a big difference. It can relieve some of the emotional burden and make you feel less alone.

Joining support groups can also be incredibly beneficial. Look for online forums or local meetups where people share similar struggles. These groups offer a sense of community and belonging. You can exchange tips, share experiences, and provide each other support. Knowing that others are going through the same challenges can be incredibly comforting. It reminds you that you're not alone in this fight. These groups often provide a safe space to express your feelings without fear of judgment.

Professional help is another critical component of a support network. Therapists and counselors can provide valuable insights and strategies for managing emotional eating. They can help you explore the underlying issues contributing to your eating habits and develop healthier coping mechanisms. Working with a therapist can give you a deeper understanding of yourself and your emotions. It's like having a guide who helps you navigate the complexities of your emotional world. Dietitians and nutritionists can also play a crucial role. They can offer practical advice on healthy eating and help you develop a balanced diet that supports your emotional and physical well-being.

Building a support network takes time and effort, but it's worth it. A strong support system can provide the emotional encouragement and accountability you need to overcome emotional eating. Whether it's friends, family, support groups, or professionals, having people who understand and support you can make a great difference in your journey toward healthier eating habits.

As we conclude this chapter on building a toolbox of coping strategies, remember that you don't have to face this alone. Each tool, from cognitive-behavioral techniques to stress management and creative outlets, can help you manage your emotions without turning to food.

CHAPTER 5

SELF-COMPASSION AND ACCEPTANCE

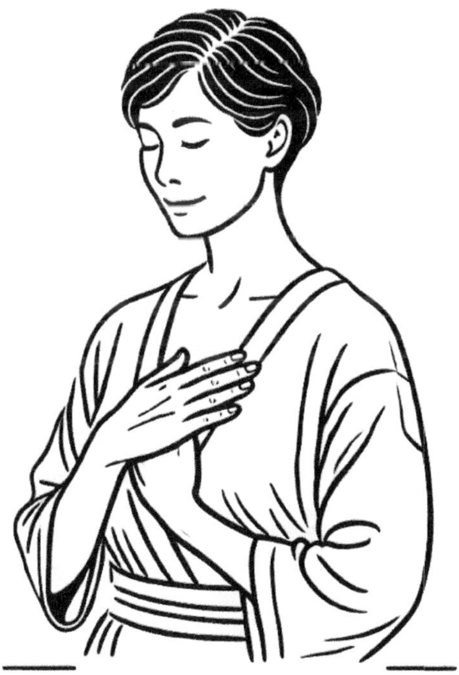

Have you ever noticed how easily you can offer a comforting word to a distressed friend but struggle to extend that kindness to yourself? Yet, when you face a similar challenge, your inner dialogue turns harsh, filled with self-criticism and blame. This chapter is about changing that narrative and learning to treat yourself with the same compassion you readily offer to others.

UNDERSTANDING SELF-COMPASSION: WHAT IT MEANS AND WHY IT MATTERS

Self-compassion is treating yourself with the same kindness, care, and understanding you would offer to a dear friend. It's about recognizing your suffering and responding with empathy rather than harsh judgment. When you practice self-compassion, you acknowledge that it's okay to be imperfect, to make mistakes, and to experience difficult emotions. You're not alone in your struggles; suffering and imperfection are part of the shared human experience.

When you approach yourself with self-compassion, you create a safe space for healing. Instead of berating yourself for eating that extra slice of cake, you acknowledge that you're human and that everyone has moments of weakness. This shift in perspective can profoundly affect your mental and emotional well-being. For instance, studies have shown that self-compassion can significantly reduce anxiety and depression. When you stop beating yourself up and offer kindness, you create a more supportive internal environment that fosters emotional resilience.

Self-compassion also enhances emotional resilience, allowing you to quickly bounce back from setbacks. Treating yourself with kindness makes you better equipped to handle life's challenges. You can see setbacks as opportunities for growth rather than personal failures. This resilience is crucial for overcoming emotional eating, as it helps you navigate the ups and downs of your journey without falling into a cycle of guilt and shame.

Another benefit of self-compassion is that it can increase motivation and personal growth. Contrary to the belief that being hard on yourself is necessary for improvement, research shows that self-compassionate individuals are more likely to take responsibility for their actions and make positive changes. You're more motivated to adopt healthy behaviors and pursue your goals when you approach yourself with kindness. You understand that you deserve care and well-being, which fuels your desire to make choices that support your long-term health.

It's important to differentiate self-compassion from self-pity and self-indulgence, as these concepts are often misunderstood. Self-compassion involves recognizing your suffering without becoming overwhelmed by it. It's about acknowledging your pain, responding with kindness, and not wallowing in it. Self-pity, on the other hand, is when you become consumed by your suffering and feel isolated in your pain. This can lead to a sense of helplessness and inaction, which is not conducive to healing.

Self-compassion is also distinct from self-indulgence. While self-compassion encourages healthy behaviors, self-indulgence involves giving in to short-term desires at the expense of long-term well-being. For example, practicing self-compassion might mean allowing yourself to rest when you're tired, while self-indulgence might mean overeating as a way to avoid dealing with difficult emotions. Self-compassion is about making choices that support your overall well-being, even if challenging.

Dr. Kristin Neff, a leading researcher in self-compassion, explains, "Self-compassion involves acting the same way towards yourself when you are having a difficult time, fail, or notice something you don't like about yourself as you would act towards a friend. Instead of just ignoring your pain with a stiff upper lip mentality, you stop to tell yourself, 'This is really difficult right now,' how can I comfort and care for myself in this moment?" Dr. Neff's research highlights the transformative power of self-compassion in fostering emotional well-being and resilience.

Findings from self-compassion studies further emphasize its importance. Research has shown that individuals who practice self-compassion experience lower stress and anxiety levels, improved emotional stability, and improved overall well-being. You create a supportive internal environment that promotes healing and growth by treating yourself with kindness and understanding.

Self-compassion is a powerful tool for overcoming emotional eating and developing a healthier relationship with yourself. By treating yourself with the same kindness and understanding you offer to others, you can reduce anxiety and depression, build emotional resilience, and foster personal growth. Embracing self-compassion allows you to navigate life's challenges with greater ease and create a more supportive internal environment for healing.

PRACTICAL EXERCISES FOR CULTIVATING SELF-COMPASSION

You're facing a stressful day at work. Deadlines are looming and you feel the weight of expectations pressing down on you. In moments like these, it's easy to fall into a cycle of self-criticism and frustration. But what if you could pause and offer yourself a moment of kindness and understanding? This is where a self-compassion break comes in. Taking a self-compassion break involves acknowledging your stress and responding with compassion. Close your eyes, take a deep breath, and say, "This is a tough moment. I'm struggling right now, and that's okay. May I be kind to myself at this moment?" This simple practice can help shift your mindset from self-criticism to self-compassion, providing you with the emotional support you need to navigate challenging situations.

Another powerful exercise is loving-kindness meditation. This practice involves sending love to yourself and others. Find a quiet place to sit comfortably and close your eyes. Begin by focusing on your breath, allowing your mind to settle. Then, silently repeat loving-kind phrases to yourself, such as "May I be happy. May I be healthy. May I be safe. May I live with ease." After a few minutes, extend these wishes to a loved one, a neutral person, and even someone you find challenging. This meditation helps cultivate a sense of compassion and connection, reducing feelings of isolation and self-judgment.

Journaling can also be a powerful tool for developing self-compassion. When you write down your thoughts and feelings, you create a space for reflection and understanding. One helpful prompt is to "write a letter to yourself from the perspective of a compassionate friend." Imagine what a supportive friend would say to you in a difficult moment. They might remind you of your strengths, offer encouragement, and reassure you that it's okay to make mistakes. Writing this letter can help you internalize these compassionate messages and shift your self-talk from critical to kind.

Another journaling prompt is to "reflect on a recent difficult experience and respond to yourself with kindness." Think about a recent challenging situation and write about how it made you feel.

Then, offer yourself words of comfort and understanding. Acknowledge that it's natural to struggle and that you deserve kindness and support. This practice can help you reframe your experiences and develop a more compassionate attitude toward yourself.

Physical gestures can also foster self-compassion. Placing a hand over your heart is a simple yet powerful gesture that can provide comfort and connection. Close your eyes, take a deep breath, and feel the warmth and pressure of your hand on your chest. This physical touch can create a sense of safety and self-soothing, reminding you that you are worthy of compassion. Another gesture is giving yourself a gentle hug. Wrap your arms around yourself and squeeze gently. This act of self-hugging can provide a sense of comfort and reassurance, helping you feel more connected to yourself.

Incorporating these self-compassion exercises into your daily life can shift how you relate to yourself. Whether it's taking a self-compassion break, practicing loving-kindness meditation, journaling, or using self-compassionate touch, these practices can help you develop a more compassionate and supportive relationship with yourself.

OVERCOMING SELF-CRITICISM: TECHNIQUES FOR BEING KINDER TO YOURSELF

Self-criticism can be sneaky and pervasive, often showing up in ways you might not even notice. Have you ever thought, "I'm so stupid for eating that," or "I'll never get this right"? These are signs of negative self-talk, a common form of self-criticism. That inner voice harshly judges and berates you, making you feel unworthy or incapable. Another sign is perfectionism—setting unrealistic standards for yourself and feeling like a failure when you don't meet them. Perfectionism can create a cycle of disappointment and self-blame, where you constantly feel like you're not good enough.

This relentless self-criticism significantly impacts emotional eating and your overall well-being. When you criticize yourself for your eating habits, it can increase feelings of shame and guilt. You might think, "I've already messed up today; I might as well keep eating." This guilt can lead to more emotional eating, creating a vicious cycle that's hard to break. Lowered self-esteem and confidence are other consequences. Constantly judging yourself harshly erodes your sense of self-worth, making it difficult to believe in your ability to make positive changes. This negativity can weigh you down, making you feel trapped in a cycle of self-doubt and emotional eating.

Cognitive restructuring can be a powerful tool for combating self-criticism. This technique involves challenging and reframing negative thoughts. When you notice a self-critical thought, ask yourself, "Is this thought accurate? What evidence do I have to support it?" Often, you'll find that these thoughts are exaggerated or unfounded. For example, if you think, "I'm terrible at managing my eating habits," challenge that by reminding yourself of times when you made healthy choices. Reframing this thought might look like, "I'm working on improving my eating habits, and I've made progress."

Practicing self-affirmations is another effective strategy. These are positive statements you repeat to yourself to counteract negative self-talk. Start by identifying areas where you feel most self-critical and create affirmations that speak to those issues. For instance, if you struggle with body image, you might say, "I appreciate my body for all it does for me." Repeat these affirmations daily, especially when you notice self-critical thoughts creeping in.

Over time, this practice can shift your mindset, helping you build a more positive self-image.

Visualization is another technique that can help reduce self-criticism. Imagine yourself as a compassionate friend. What would this friend say to you in moments of self-doubt or criticism? Visualize offering yourself the exact words of kindness and support. This exercise can create a sense of emotional distance from your self-critical thoughts, making responding with compassion rather than judgment easier. By seeing yourself through the eyes of a compassionate friend, you can soften your inner dialogue and nurture a more supportive relationship with yourself.

By recognizing the signs of self-criticism and implementing these techniques, you can foster self-kindness and reduce the negative impact of self-judgment. Cognitive restructuring, self-affirmations, and visualization can help you challenge and reframe your self-critical thoughts, creating a more supportive and compassionate inner dialogue. Remember, being kinder to yourself is not about ignoring your struggles but about responding to them with understanding and empathy.

EMBRACING IMPERFECTION: PROGRESS OVER PERFECTION

Have you ever found yourself stuck in the pursuit of perfection, only to end up feeling more frustrated and defeated? Embracing imperfection is a transformative approach, especially when dealing with emotional eating. Mistakes and setbacks are inevitable. They are not signs of failure but rather opportunities for growth and learning. Accepting that imperfection is a natural part of life opens the door to understanding and self-compassion. Through these experiences, you learn more about yourself and what strategies work best for you.

Perfectionism, on the other hand, can be a significant barrier to progress. When you strive for perfection, you set yourself up for an all-or-nothing mindset. You might feel it's not worth doing if you can't do something perfectly. This kind of thinking can be detrimental. For example, if you aim to eat perfectly healthy and then slip up, you might think, "I've already ruined my diet, so I might as well keep eating." This can lead to binge eating and further emotional distress. Perfectionism also fosters a fear of failure, making you avoid challenges that could lead to growth. You might hesitate to try new coping mechanisms or attend support groups because you're afraid of not doing them perfectly.

Focusing on progress rather than perfection can be liberating. Celebrate small victories and incremental improvements. These small steps add up over time and lead to significant changes. Setting realistic and achievable goals is crucial. Instead of aiming to eliminate emotional eating overnight, start with manageable steps like keeping a food journal or practicing mindful eating once a day. Reflecting on your personal growth and milestones can also be motivating. Take time to acknowledge your achievements, even if the progress seems small. Each step forward is a step in the right direction.

Embracing imperfection means understanding that setbacks are not failures but opportunities for growth. It's about recognizing that progress is made through small, consistent steps rather than grand, perfect gestures. When you focus on progress, you create a more supportive and compassionate environment for yourself. You learn to celebrate your achievements, no matter how small, and use setbacks as learning experiences.

REAL-LIFE STORIES OF SELF-COMPASSION IN ACTION

Maria's Story

Meet Maria, a woman who struggled with emotional eating for years. Maria often found herself turning to food when she felt overwhelmed or stressed. She would binge on snacks late at night, only to wake up feeling guilty and ashamed. This cycle took a toll on her mental and physical health. One day, Maria stumbled upon the concept of self-kindness. She decided to try it, though she was initially skeptical.

Maria began by practicing self-compassion breaks during moments of stress. Whenever she felt the urge to eat emotionally, she paused, took a deep breath, and told herself, "This is a tough moment, and that's okay. I deserve kindness right now." These simple words had a profound impact on her. Gradually, Maria noticed that her cravings lessened, and she started to develop healthier coping mechanisms. Her journey wasn't easy—there were days when she reverted to old habits. But with persistence, Maria learned to treat herself with the same kindness she offered to others. Over time, she saw significant improvements in her mental and emotional well-being, and her relationship with food became much healthier.

Jake's Story

Jake worked a high-pressure job that often left him feeling frazzled and tense. To cope, he would eat large amounts of junk food, hoping to numb his stress. This only led to weight gain and a sense of helplessness. One day, Jake decided to try something different. He incorporated loving-kindness meditation into his daily routine. He spent a few minutes sending compassionate thoughts to himself and others each morning. He would say, "May I be happy. May I be healthy. May I live with ease."

This practice helped Jake cultivate a sense of inner peace and reduced his reliance on food to manage stress. The changes took time. Jake faced many challenges, including initial resistance to the idea of self-compassion. But he persisted, and over time, he found that his anxiety levels decreased. He became more resilient and better equipped to handle the pressures of his job. The positive changes also extended to his physical health—Jake lost weight and felt more energetic.

Developing self-compassion is a process that requires patience and effort. Both Maria and Jake faced initial struggles and challenges. Maria found it difficult to break the cycle of emotional eating, while Jake was skeptical about the effectiveness of self-compassion. However, they both discovered techniques and practices that worked for them. Maria found self-compassion breaks to be incredibly effective, while Jake benefited from loving-kindness meditation. These practices helped them develop a kinder, more understanding relationship with themselves.

The outcomes of practicing self-compassion are profound. For Maria, embracing self-kindness led to improved mental and emotional well-being. She no longer felt trapped in a cycle of guilt and shame. Instead, she developed healthier coping mechanisms and a more balanced relationship with food. Jake experienced similar benefits. His anxiety levels decreased, and he became more resilient. He felt more at peace with himself and was able to manage stress without turning to food. Both Maria and Jake also noticed improvements in their physical health. Maria lost weight and felt more energetic, while Jake experienced better overall health and well-being.

These stories offer inspirational takeaways for anyone struggling with emotional eating. The journeys of Maria and Jake show that self-compassion can transform your life. It requires patience and persistence, but the benefits are worth the effort. By treating yourself with kindness and understanding, you can improve your mental and emotional well-being, develop a healthier relationship with food, and enhance your overall quality of life. Remember, self-compassion is not about being perfect. It's about recognizing your struggles and responding with empathy and care. The power of self-compassion lies in its ability to foster healing and growth, helping you navigate life's challenges with greater ease and resilience.

In this chapter, we've explored the transformative power of self-compassion and how it can help you overcome emotional eating. By practicing self-kindness, you can improve your mental and emotional well-being, develop healthier coping mechanisms, and build a more positive relationship with yourself.

Hi there!

Thank you for sticking around! I hope you have enjoyed the book so far and are ready to try out some of the new things you have learned.

Your opinion really matters to me, and I'd love to hear what you think about the book. Could you please take a few minutes to write a review? Your review helps others decide if this book is right for them, and it helps me make future books even better.

Here's how you can leave a review:

1. **Go to the Book's Page**: Visit the website where you bought or read this book.
2. **Find the Review Section**: Scroll down to where you can leave a comment or rating.
3. **Share Your Thoughts**: Write a little about what you liked. Did you learn something new? What part was your favorite?

Your review doesn't have to be lengthy—just a few sentences can make a big difference. Whether you loved the book or have ideas about improving it, I appreciate your honest feedback.

Thank you so much for your time and support!

Best wishes,

Lawrence E. Meadows

Author of "Triumph Over Emotional Eating"

CHAPTER 6

THE ROLE OF SOCIETY AND MEDIA

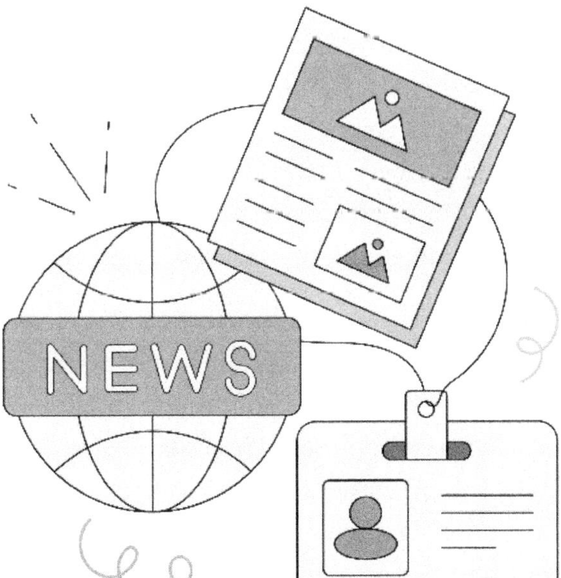

Picture waking up and scrolling through your social media feed first thing in the morning. Influencers flaunt their toned bodies and share snippets of their latest diet plans. Later in the day, you flip through a magazine at the doctor's office, and the cover promises a "miracle weight loss" solution that will transform your body in two weeks. Messages like these are everywhere, subtly shaping our beliefs and actions about food, body image, and self-worth. It's no wonder that navigating the world of diet culture can feel overwhelming and disheartening.

MEDIA MESSAGES: DECODING DIET CULTURE

Diet culture is pervasive, infiltrating various media channels and influencing how we perceive ourselves and our eating habits. Advertisements promoting weight loss products are a common sight. Turn on the TV or browse the internet, and you'll encounter ads selling diet pills, detox teas, and meal replacement shakes, all promising quick fixes to achieve the "ideal" body. These advertisements often feature before-and-after photos, highlighting dramatic transformations that seem too good to be true. They prey on our insecurities, convincing us we need these products to be happy and accepted.

Social media influencers play a significant role in perpetuating diet culture. With millions of followers, influencers often endorse fad diets and extreme fitness routines. They share their "secret" tips for losing weight, often without scientific backing. Influencers post curated images of their meals, workouts, and slim physiques, creating an illusion of perfection. This can make you feel like you need to follow their advice to fit in or achieve similar results. The constant exposure to these messages can lead to unhealthy comparisons and a skewed perception of what it means to be healthy.

TV shows and movies also glorify thinness, reinforcing the idea that being slim is synonymous with success, beauty, and happiness. Thin characters are often portrayed as attractive, successful, and desirable. At the same time, those with larger bodies are depicted as lazy, unattractive, or in need of transformation. This representation can profoundly impact our self-esteem and how we view our bodies. When thinness is constantly celebrated, and larger bodies are stigmatized, it can lead to internalized beliefs that our worth is tied to our appearance.

The impact of diet culture on eating habits is significant. Exposure to these messages can increase anxiety around eating, making you constantly question your food choices. You might worry about every calorie, scrutinize nutrition labels, and feel guilty for indulging in certain foods. This anxiety can lead to the adoption of restrictive eating patterns, where you eliminate entire food groups or severely limit your intake in an attempt to achieve the "ideal" body. Restrictive eating can be harmful, leading to nutrient deficiencies, decreased energy levels, and a strained relationship with food.

Diet culture also normalizes unhealthy dieting behaviors. It promotes the idea that extreme measures like skipping meals, juice cleanses, and detox diets are necessary for weight loss. These behaviors are often framed as acts of discipline and self-control when, in reality, they can be detrimental to your physical and mental health. Normalizing these behaviors can make it challenging to recognize when you're engaging in unhealthy practices, as society often celebrates and encourages them.

Examples of diet culture messaging are abundant and varied. Magazine covers frequently feature headlines like "Lose 10 Pounds in 10 Days!" or "Get a Bikini Body Fast!" These messages promise quick results and reinforce the idea that our bodies need constant improvement. On Instagram, you might come across posts showcasing extreme before-and-after photos. Influencers share their weight loss journeys, emphasizing how much happier and more confident they feel after losing weight. These posts can create unrealistic expectations and make you feel inadequate if you don't achieve similar results.

Weight loss challenges trending on TikTok are another example. These challenges often promote rapid weight loss through extreme diets or intense exercise routines. Participants share their progress and encourage others to join, creating a competitive environment that can be harmful. The pressure to participate and achieve the same results can lead to disordered eating and an unhealthy obsession with weight loss.

To navigate these messages, it's essential to critically evaluate the media you consume. Start by asking critical questions about the source and intent of the message. Who is promoting this product or diet, and what do they stand to gain? Are they qualified to give nutritional advice? Examining the scientific validity of diet claims is crucial. Many fad diets lack scientific backing and can be harmful. Look for evidence-based information from reputable sources like registered dietitians or healthcare professionals.

Recognizing signs of unrealistic body standards can help you question and resist diet culture narratives. Pay attention to heavily edited images or portray an unattainable level of perfection. Remember that everyone's body is different, and there is no singular approach to health. By developing a critical eye and questioning the messages you encounter, you can protect yourself from the negative impact of diet culture and foster a healthier relationship with food and your body.

SOCIETAL PRESSURES: THE IMPACT OF BEAUTY STANDARDS

Beauty standards have been influencing how we see ourselves for centuries. During the Renaissance, for example, curvaceous figures were celebrated. Paintings often depicted fuller-bodied women as symbols of fertility and wealth. Fast forward to the 1920s, and the flapper era ushered in a preference for slim, boyish figures. Each era brought its own ideal, and people often went to great lengths to conform to these changing standards.

Different cultures have also held unique beauty ideals. In some African cultures, fuller bodies were considered beautiful and a sign of prosperity. In contrast, many Asian cultures valued petite and slender figures. These cultural shifts show how fluid beauty standards can be, but they also highlight the pressure to conform to societal expectations. The impact of these evolving standards is far-reaching, affecting people's self-esteem and body image.

Society and media heavily shape today's beauty standards, creating a complicated landscape. The "slim-thick" phenomenon, for example, has become increasingly popular. This ideal emphasizes a slim waist paired with curvy hips and a large bust, a combination that is naturally rare and difficult to achieve. Celebrity culture also plays a significant role in shaping these ideals. Celebrities like Kim Kardashian and Kylie Jenner have popularized this body type, leading many to pursue extreme measures to emulate it.

The fashion and beauty industries further perpetuate these ideals. Models with specific body types dominate runways and magazine covers, reinforcing the notion that only specific shapes are beautiful. Fashion brands often design clothes for smaller sizes, making it challenging for people with diverse body types to find flattering options. Beauty products are marketed with the promise of achieving flawless skin and a perfect figure, feeding into the desire to meet these unattainable standards.

These societal pressures have a profound impact on self-esteem and body image. Exposure to narrow beauty ideals can lead to increased body dissatisfaction. You might find yourself comparing your body to those you see in magazines or on social media, feeling inadequate or unattractive. This constant comparison can create a sense of worthlessness and drive you to engage in unhealthy behaviors to conform to these ideals.

The pressure to meet unattainable beauty standards can also lead to negative self-body talk. You might criticize yourself for not fitting into a particular mold, focusing on perceived flaws rather than appreciating your unique attributes. This negative self-talk can damage your self-esteem and contribute to a cycle of shame and self-loathing. The societal emphasis on appearance can make it challenging to develop a positive self-image and appreciate your body for what it can do rather than how it looks.

Intersectionality plays a crucial role in understanding the impact of beauty standards. Non-Eurocentric beauty traits are often marginalized, leading to a lack of representation and validation for people of color. For instance, media and fashion often favor lighter skin tones, straight hair, and slim noses, sidelining the diverse beauty of different ethnicities. This marginalization can make it challenging for individuals with non-Eurocentric features to feel beautiful and accepted.

Socioeconomic status also plays a role in accessing beauty treatments and achieving societal ideals. High-fashion clothes, cosmetic procedures, and premium beauty products often have hefty price tags. Those with limited financial resources may feel excluded from the beauty standards set by society, reinforcing feelings of inadequacy and marginalization.

CHALLENGING UNHEALTHY NORMS: BUILDING A POSITIVE BODY IMAGE

Embracing body positivity and self-acceptance can feel like a radical act in a society that constantly tells you to change. But it's essential for building a healthier relationship with yourself. Body positivity is about embracing body diversity and celebrating all shapes and sizes. It means recognizing that beauty isn't confined to a narrow standard but is expansive and inclusive. Honoring your body as it is, flaws and all, can be liberating and empowering.

Start by practicing positive self-talk and affirmations to foster a positive body image. The way you speak to yourself matters. Replace negative thoughts with affirmations that celebrate your strengths and unique qualities. Instead of focusing on what you perceive as flaws, highlight what you love about yourself. Look in the mirror and say, "I am strong," or "I am beautiful just as I am." These affirmations can shift your mindset, helping you build a more positive self-image.

Engage in body-positive activities that promote acceptance and appreciation. Practices like body-positive yoga focus on how you feel rather than look. These classes emphasize inclusivity and self-love, creating a supportive environment where you can move your body without judgment. Activities like dancing, swimming, or hiking can also be joyous ways to connect with your body and appreciate its capabilities. The goal is to find activities that make you feel good, both physically and mentally.

Surrounding yourself with supportive and accepting communities can make a significant difference. Join groups or online communities that promote body positivity and self-acceptance. These spaces can provide encouragement, understanding, and validation.

Being part of a community that celebrates diversity and challenges societal norms can reinforce your journey toward self-acceptance. It's easier to embrace your body when you see others doing the same and realize you're not alone in your struggles.

Self-compassion plays a crucial role in improving body image. Treating yourself with kindness and understanding can reduce self-criticism and foster a more positive relationship with your body. When you engage in negative self-talk, pause and reframe those thoughts with compassion. Ask yourself, "Would I say this to a friend?" If the answer is no, then it's not something you should say to yourself, either. Replace harsh judgments with compassionate thoughts that acknowledge your worth and humanity.

Building a positive body image is an ongoing process that requires effort and commitment. Strategies that can help include practicing positive self-talk, engaging in body-positive activities, surrounding yourself with supportive communities, and cultivating self-compassion. Challenging unhealthy norms and embracing body diversity can foster a more positive and accepting relationship with your body.

STRATEGIES FOR MEDIA LITERACY: CURATING YOUR FEED

In today's digital age, media literacy is more important than ever. Media literacy is about understanding the influence of media on your perceptions and behaviors. It involves developing critical thinking skills to analyze media messages so you can make informed decisions about what to believe and how to act. You're constantly bombarded with information when you scroll through social media, watch TV, or read articles online. Some of it can be helpful, but many can be misleading or harmful. Understanding how media shapes your thoughts and actions is the first step in taking control of your media consumption.

One of the most effective ways to foster media literacy is by curating a positive social media feed. Start by following body-positive influencers and accounts that promote self-acceptance and diversity. These accounts counterbalance the pervasive diet culture and unrealistic beauty standards often seen online. They showcase natural, unedited bodies and celebrate all shapes and sizes, reminding you that beauty is diverse and multifaceted.

Conversely, it's crucial to unfollow or mute accounts that promote diet culture. If you notice an account constantly pushing fad diets, weight loss products, or unrealistic body standards, it might be time to hit that unfollow button. Removing these negative influences can help reduce the pressure to conform to harmful ideals. Instead, fill your feed with content that supports your mental and emotional well-being. Follow accounts that focus on mental health, self-care, and holistic well-being. Engaging with uplifting and supportive content can inspire you to cultivate a healthier relationship with yourself and your body.

Recognizing and resisting harmful media messages requires a keen eye and a critical mindset. Start by fact-checking information and claims you come across. If an influencer promotes a diet that promises rapid weight loss, take a moment to research its validity. Check credible sources like registered dietitians or scientific studies. Many fad diets lack scientific backing and can be harmful, so it's essential to seek evidence-based information.

Using tools and apps to filter content can also be beneficial. Social media detox apps can help you manage your screen time and reduce exposure to negative content. These apps allow you to limit how long you spend on social media and even block certain types of content. You can create a healthier and more positive online environment by taking control of your media consumption.

Expert insights on media literacy can provide valuable guidance. Media studies scholars often emphasize the importance of critical thinking and media literacy education. Dr. Renee Hobbs, a leading expert in media literacy, states, "Media literacy is about understanding how media shapes our perceptions and behaviors. Developing critical thinking skills enables us to navigate the media landscape more effectively and make informed decisions."

Research findings support the positive impact of media literacy education. A study published in the "Journal of Media Literacy Education" found that individuals who received media literacy training were better equipped to identify and resist harmful media messages. They reported lower levels of body dissatisfaction and were less likely to engage in unhealthy dieting behaviors. These findings highlight the importance of media literacy in promoting mental and emotional well-being.

Developing media literacy is an ongoing process that requires practice and vigilance. By understanding the influence of media, curating a positive feed, and critically evaluating media messages, you can take control of your media consumption. This protects you from harmful influences and empowers you to create a supportive and uplifting online environment.

OVERCOMING SOCIETAL PRESSURES

Rebecca's Story

Meet Rebecca, a young woman who always felt she was at odds with society's beauty standards. Growing up, she was bombarded with images of ultra-thin models and actresses, which led her to believe that her naturally curvy body was something to be ashamed of. Rebecca spent years trying to conform to these standards, engaging in restrictive diets and excessive exercise routines that left her physically and emotionally drained.

One day, after yet another failed diet, Rebecca decided she'd had enough. She researched body positivity and stumbled upon communities that celebrated all body types. Inspired, Rebecca began to engage in body-positive activism, attending events and joining online forums where she met like-minded individuals. She found solace and strength in their shared experiences, and slowly, her perspective began to shift. She started practicing mindfulness and self-compassion, learning to appreciate her body for what it could do rather than how it looked.

The journey wasn't easy—Rebecca faced negative comments and criticism, especially on social media, but she persisted. Today, Rebecca feels more confident and at peace with her body.

Tom's Story

Meet Tom, who spent most of his life battling his weight. Tom grew up in a household where thinness was equated with success, and he internalized these beliefs. He tried every fad diet under the sun, from juice cleanses to low-carb regimes, but nothing seemed to work long-term. The constant cycle of losing and gaining weight took a toll on his mental health. One day, Tom attended a workshop on mindful eating and realized that his relationship with food was deeply unhealthy. He resisted diet culture and focused on finding a healthier relationship with food.

Tom joined a local support group where he met people who were also seeking to break free from the shackles of diet culture. They shared tips, offered support, and held each other accountable. Tom started practicing mindfulness during meals, savoring each bite and paying attention to his hunger and fullness cues. He also incorporated self-compassion exercises into his daily routine, reminding himself that his worth wasn't tied to his weight.

The road was filled with challenges—Tom struggled with social media pressure and the temptation to revert to old habits. However, with his new community's support and commitment to mindfulness, Tom found a balanced and mindful approach to eating. He feels happier and healthier mentally and physically and enjoys a more positive relationship with food.

Lisa's Story

Meet Lisa, a teenager who faced immense pressure to conform to beauty standards perpetuated by her peers and media. Lisa constantly compared herself to others, feeling inadequate and unattractive. She took a stand against these societal pressures by engaging in body-positive activism. Lisa started a blog sharing her struggles and triumphs, advocating for self-acceptance and challenging the unrealistic beauty standards that plagued her generation.

Her blog gained traction, and she built a community of followers who resonated with her message. Lisa also sought support from like-minded communities, joining groups that promoted body positivity and self-love. She practiced mindfulness and self-compassion, learning to gracefully navigate negative comments and criticism. Despite the challenges, Lisa's activism and self-compassion practices significantly improved her mental and emotional well-being. She gained confidence and self-esteem, and her approach to eating became more balanced and mindful. Lisa's story is a testament to the power of resisting societal pressures and embracing self-acceptance.

Real-life stories like those of Rebecca, Tom, and Lisa highlight the transformative power of challenging societal pressures and embracing self-acceptance. These individuals employed various strategies, from body-positive activism and seeking supportive communities to practicing mindfulness and self-compassion. They faced numerous obstacles, including social media pressure and negative comments, but their perseverance led to improved mental and emotional well-being, greater confidence, and a more balanced approach to eating. These stories inspire, showing that overcoming societal pressures and developing a healthier relationship with oneself and food is possible. You can take steps towards a healthier and more fulfilling life by understanding and addressing the societal pressures related to body image and eating habits.

CHAPTER 7

DEVELOPING A HOLISTIC APPROACH TO WELL-BEING

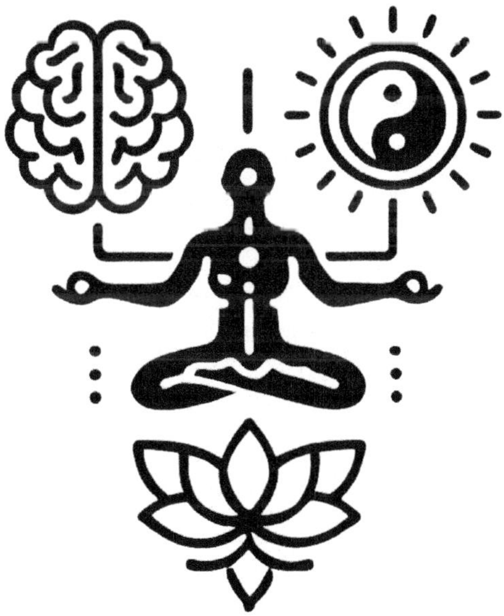

Have you ever felt like you're juggling too many balls at once, struggling to keep them all in the air? One moment, you're trying to eat healthier; the next, you're stressing about work deadlines, and in between, you're squeezing in a few minutes of exercise. It's exhausting. Often, emotional eating sneaks in when we're overwhelmed, and it's in these moments that a holistic approach to well-being can make all the difference. Addressing the interconnectedness of your mind, body, and spirit can help you find balance and reduce the reliance on food as an emotional crutch.

THE INTERCONNECTEDNESS OF MIND, BODY, AND SPIRIT

Holistic health is about understanding that your emotional, physical, and mental health are deeply intertwined. When one aspect is out of balance, it can affect the others. For instance, if you're emotionally distressed, it can manifest physically through headaches or digestive issues. Likewise, poor physical health can dampen your mood and lead to negative thought patterns. Recognizing this interconnectedness allows you to address emotional eating from multiple angles, creating a more comprehensive and practical approach.

Your emotional well-being has a profound impact on your physical health. When you're stressed or anxious, your body releases cortisol, which can lead to weight gain, especially around the abdomen. Chronic stress can also weaken your immune system, making you more susceptible to illnesses. By managing your emotions through techniques like mindfulness and stress reduction, you can improve your physical health and reduce the triggers for emotional eating.

Mental health plays a crucial role in fostering a positive body image. When you're mentally resilient, you're better equipped to challenge negative thoughts about your body and develop a more compassionate view of yourself. This mental strength can prevent the cycle of self-criticism that often leads to emotional eating. For example, practicing cognitive-behavioral techniques to reframe negative thoughts can help you build a healthier, more positive body image. Feeling good about yourself makes you less likely to use food to cope with negative emotions.

Physical health, in turn, influences your emotional and mental states. Regular exercise releases endorphins, which are natural mood lifters. Physical activity can help reduce stress, anxiety, and depression, making you less likely to turn to food for comfort. Maintaining a balanced diet can also stabilize your blood sugar levels, preventing mood swings that might trigger emotional eating. Imagine the difference between starting your day with a nutritious breakfast versus skipping it and feeling irritable and tired by mid-morning. These small changes can have a significant impact on your overall well-being.

Balance is critical to holistic health. Avoid extremes in diet and exercise because they can lead to burnout and make emotional eating more likely. Strive for moderation and flexibility. Find harmony between work, rest, and play to create a well-rounded and sustainable lifestyle. For example, if your workday is particularly demanding, ensure you carve out time for relaxation in the evening, whether reading a book, taking a bath, or practicing mindfulness.

Spiritual practices can also contribute significantly to your overall well-being. Meditation and mindfulness practices help you stay present and aware, reducing the tendency to eat mindlessly. Connecting with nature can provide peace and grounding, allowing you to reset and recharge. Engaging in community and acts of service can foster a sense of belonging and purpose, which are crucial for emotional health. Volunteering at a local shelter or participating in community activities can provide fulfillment and reduce feelings of isolation.

PRACTICAL TIPS FOR HOLISTIC HEALTH

Start a daily gratitude practice. Spend a few minutes each day reflecting on things you're grateful for. This simple act can shift your focus from what's lacking to what's abundant in your life, improving your emotional well-being. Incorporate gentle stretching or yoga into your routine to reduce physical tension and promote relaxation. Set aside time for self-reflection and meditation. Even just five minutes a day can make a significant difference in your mental clarity and emotional resilience.

Integrating these practices into your daily life can create a balanced approach to health and well-being. This holistic perspective helps you address the root causes of emotional eating, leading to more sustainable and fulfilling changes. Remember, it's not about perfection but making small, consistent steps towards a healthier, more balanced life.

NUTRITION AND NOURISHMENT: EATING FOR HEALTH AND HAPPINESS

The food you eat plays a crucial role in how you feel physically and emotionally. Balanced nutrition is more than just managing your weight; it's about providing your body with the nutrients it needs to function optimally. A balanced diet includes a variety of nutrients, each playing a unique role in your overall health.

- Proteins, carbohydrates, and fats—known as macronutrients—are the building blocks of your diet. Proteins are essential for muscle repair and growth, carbohydrates provide energy, and fats support brain health and hormone production.
- Micronutrients, including vitamins and minerals, are equally essential. Vitamins like A, C, and E are antioxidants that protect your cells from damage. B vitamins support energy production and brain function. Minerals such as calcium and magnesium are vital for bone health and muscle function.

When you consume a diet rich in various nutrients, you're fueling your body with what it needs to thrive. Consider colorful fruits, vegetables, lean proteins, whole grains, and healthy fats like avocados and nuts. These foods provide a spectrum of nutrients that support your overall well-being.

What you eat profoundly affects your mood and emotional well-being. Foods that boost serotonin levels, like those rich in tryptophan (found in turkey, eggs, and cheese), can enhance mood and promote happiness. On the other hand, sugar and processed foods can lead to mood swings and energy crashes. While they might provide a quick boost, the subsequent dip in blood sugar can leave you feeling irritable and tired. It's like riding a roller coaster of emotions, where the highs are fleeting, and the lows can be pretty challenging. Consider how you feel after indulging in a sugary snack compared to a balanced meal. The difference is often stark.

Maintaining a balanced and nourishing diet requires some planning and mindfulness. Start by planning balanced meals that include all the macronutrients and a variety of micronutrients. Aim to fill half your plate with colorful vegetables, a quarter with lean protein, and the remaining quarter with whole grains or starchy vegetables. Incorporate whole foods into your diet, such as fresh fruits, vegetables, whole grains, and nuts. These foods are nutrient-dense and provide sustained energy. Avoid restrictive diets that eliminate entire food groups, as they can lead to nutrient deficiencies and feelings of deprivation. Instead, focus on intuitive eating—listening to your body's hunger and fullness cues.

Focusing on balanced nutrition can improve your mood, energy levels, and overall health. Remember, it's not about perfection but about making mindful choices that nourish your body and support your well-being. Balancing your diet with various nutrients helps you feel your best, making it easier to manage emotional eating and enjoy a healthier, happier life.

SLEEP AND STRESS: HOW REST AFFECTS EATING HABITS

Sleep is more than just a time for your body to rest; it plays a crucial role in your overall health, affecting everything from hormone regulation to cognitive function. When you don't get enough sleep, your body's production of hormones like ghrelin and leptin gets disrupted. Ghrelin, the "hunger hormone," increases, making you hungrier, while leptin, which signals fullness, decreases. This imbalance can increase cravings for high-calorie, sugary foods, setting the stage for emotional eating.

Sleep also impacts your cognitive function and mood. A lack of sleep can impair your ability to think clearly, make decisions, and manage stress. When you're sleep-deprived, you're more likely to feel irritable, anxious, and depressed. These negative emotions can drive you to seek comfort in food, particularly those high in sugar and fat. It's a vicious cycle: poor sleep leads to poor food choices, which can further disrupt your sleep, creating a loop that's hard to break. For instance, after a sleepless night, you might reach for that extra cup of coffee and a donut to get through the day, only to crash later and disrupt your sleep again.

The connection between sleep and eating habits is undeniable. Your body's natural hunger and satiety signals get thrown off when you're tired. You might eat more than usual because your body is trying to compensate for the lack of energy. Poor sleep can also increase cortisol levels, the stress hormone, which further fuels cravings for high-calorie foods. After a restless night, you're more inclined to snack throughout the day, seeking quick energy boosts to combat fatigue. This can lead to a pattern of emotional eating, where food becomes a coping mechanism for stress and tiredness.

Improving your sleep quality can profoundly impact your overall well-being and help reduce emotional eating. Start by creating a bedtime routine that signals your body that it's time to wind down. Try to go to bed and wake up at the same time every day, even on weekends. Reducing screen time before bed can also improve sleep quality. The blue light emitted by electronics can interfere with your body's natural sleep-wake cycle. Consider reading a book, taking a warm bath, or practicing relaxation techniques instead. Optimizing your sleep environment is another key factor. Keep your bedroom cool, dark, and quiet. Investing in a comfortable mattress and pillow can also make a significant difference.

Managing stress is another crucial aspect of improving sleep and reducing emotional eating. Practicing relaxation techniques before bed, such as deep breathing exercises or progressive muscle relaxation, can help calm your mind and prepare your body for sleep. Journaling before bed can also be a helpful tool. Write down any worries or thoughts keeping you awake, then set them aside for the night. Meditation is another effective stress management tool.

Even a few minutes of mindfulness meditation daily can help reduce stress and improve sleep quality. If stress consistently interferes with your sleep and eating habits, seeking professional help might be beneficial. A therapist can provide strategies and support to help you manage stress more effectively.

Improving your sleep and managing stress can create a positive ripple effect on your eating habits and overall well-being. Adequate sleep helps regulate your hormones, improves your mood, and enhances your cognitive function, making it easier to make healthier food choices. Reducing stress can also help break the cycle of emotional eating, allowing you to find healthier ways to cope with life's challenges.

PHYSICAL ACTIVITY: MOVING FOR JOY, NOT PUNISHMENT

Imagine stepping onto a dance floor, feeling the beat of the music pulse through your veins, and letting your body move freely. Or picture yourself hiking up a scenic trail, the fresh air filling your lungs, and the beauty of nature surrounding you. These are moments of joy; physical activity can be about finding that joy rather than punishing yourself for what you ate. Exercise should feel good, not like a chore. It's about discovering what makes you feel alive and happy. Exploring different types of exercise can be an excellent way to find what you love.

- Dancing, whether salsa, hip-hop, or even a Zumba class, is a fantastic option. The rhythm, the movement, and the energy can lift your spirits and make you forget you're exercising.

- Hiking offers a different kind of joy. It's a chance to connect with nature, enjoy the serenity of the outdoors, and challenge your body in a way that feels invigorating.
- Swimming is another option that combines physical exertion with a sense of weightlessness and freedom. The water can be incredibly soothing, providing a full-body workout without the strain on your joints.
- Joining group fitness classes or sports teams can add a social element to your exercise routine. Something is motivating about working out with others, sharing the experience, and supporting each other. Group classes like yoga, spinning, or kickboxing provide structure and community. Sports teams offer camaraderie and the thrill of competition, whether it's a friendly game of soccer, volleyball, or basketball. The key is finding activities you genuinely enjoy, making exercise a positive and enjoyable experience.

Physical activity has profound mental and emotional benefits. When you exercise, your body releases endorphins, often called "feel-good" chemicals. These endorphins interact with receptors in your brain, reducing pain perception and triggering positive feelings. It's like a natural high that can improve mood and reduce stress. Regular exercise can also boost your self-esteem and body image. When you engage in physical activity, you start appreciating what your body can do rather than just how it looks. This shift in focus can foster a healthier, more positive relationship with your body.

Integrating movement into your daily life doesn't have to be complicated. Start with small, manageable changes. Walking or biking to work is a great way to incorporate exercise into your routine without taking extra time out of your day. If that's not feasible, consider parking farther away from your destination or using the stairs instead of the elevator. Taking short movement breaks throughout the day can also make a big difference. Stand up, stretch, quickly walk around the block, or do light exercises like squats or lunges for a few minutes. These breaks can refresh your mind and body, making you more productive and less likely to reach for snacks out of boredom or stress.

Involving family or friends in your exercise plans can add an element of fun and accountability. Plan weekend hikes, join a local sports league, or schedule regular workout sessions with a friend. The social interaction makes the activity more enjoyable and provides support and motivation. Sharing these experiences with loved ones can strengthen relationships and create positive memories associated with physical activity.

Finding joy in movement is about discovering what resonates with you. It's about making exercise a celebration of what your body can do rather than a punishment for what you ate. Embrace activities that make you feel good and let the joy of movement guide you towards a healthier, happier life.

CREATING A BALANCED LIFESTYLE: DAILY ROUTINES FOR WELL-BEING

A balanced lifestyle begins with establishing daily routines that promote overall health and help reduce emotional eating. Consistency is vital to creating healthy habits. When you follow a routine, your body and mind know what to expect, reducing the chaos that can lead to stress and emotional eating. Think about how much smoother your day runs when you start with a clear plan. It's this kind of structure that can make all the difference.

Balancing work, rest, and leisure activities is crucial for maintaining a healthy lifestyle. It's easy to get caught up in the hustle and forget to take breaks or make time for the things you love. Overworking yourself can lead to burnout, making you more likely to turn to food for comfort. On the other hand, neglecting your responsibilities can lead to stress and anxiety, which can also trigger emotional eating. Finding that sweet spot where you can comfortably juggle work, rest, and play is vital for your well-being.

Consider starting your day with a morning routine that sets a positive tone. This could include stretching, a short walk, or even just enjoying a quiet cup of coffee while reflecting on your goals for the day. This peaceful start can create a more productive and less stressful day. In the evening, establish routines that promote relaxation and restful sleep. This might involve winding down with a good book, taking a warm bath, or practicing gentle yoga stretches. These activities signal to your body that it's time to relax and prepare for sleep, helping you unwind and reducing the likelihood of late-night snacking.

Midday routines are just as crucial for maintaining energy and focus. Consider incorporating short breaks throughout your workday to stretch, walk, or practice deep breathing exercises. These breaks can refresh your mind and body, making you more productive and less likely to experience the afternoon slump that often leads to unhealthy snacking. Keep healthy snacks on hand to nourish your body and maintain steady energy levels throughout the day.

Self-care is an essential component of a balanced lifestyle. It's not just about pampering yourself; it's about taking deliberate steps to nurture your well-being. Set aside time for hobbies and relaxation activities that bring you joy and help you recharge. Whether painting, gardening, or playing a musical instrument, engaging in these activities can provide a much-needed break from the daily grind and reduce stress levels. Practicing mindfulness and stress reduction techniques, such as meditation or deep breathing exercises, can also support your well-being by helping you stay present and calm in the face of life's challenges.

Practical tools and strategies make it easier to maintain these balanced routines. Using planners or apps to schedule self-care activities ensures you prioritize your well-being amidst your busy schedule. Set realistic and achievable goals for your health and well-being, breaking them down into manageable steps. For example, if you want to incorporate more physical activity into your day, start with a 10-minute walk and gradually increase the time as you build the habit. Regularly reviewing and adjusting your routines is also important. Life is dynamic, and your routines should be flexible enough to adapt to changes while supporting your overall well-being.

Incorporating these practices into your daily life can help you create a balanced lifestyle that supports your physical, emotional, and mental health. By establishing consistent routines, balancing work and leisure, and prioritizing self-care, you can reduce the triggers for emotional eating and build a foundation for long-term well-being.

Remember, it's about progress, not perfection. Small, consistent steps can significantly improve your overall health and happiness, making it easier to manage emotional eating and enjoy a more fulfilling life.

CHAPTER 8

PERSONAL STORIES OF STRUGGLE AND RECOVERY

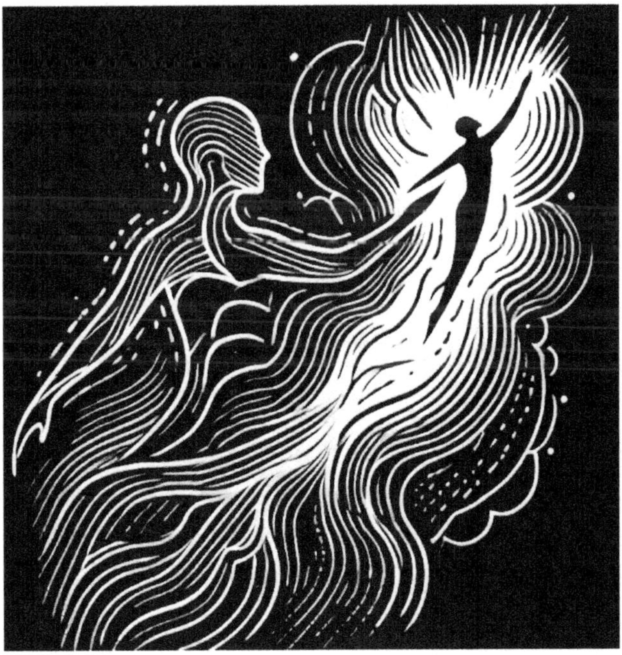

OVERCOMING EMOTIONAL EATING: SARAH'S JOURNEY

Sarah grew up in a family where food was more than just nourishment; it was a source of comfort, celebration, and, sometimes, a coping mechanism. Her parents often used food as a way to reward or console her, which laid the foundation for her emotional eating habits. Family gatherings were always centered around lavish meals, and any emotional distress was quickly met with a treat or a hearty dish. This pattern continued into her adult life, shaping her relationship with food in ways she didn't fully understand until much later.

As Sarah entered the corporate world, she quickly climbed the ladder, landing a high-stress job in a fast-paced industry. The demands of her career were relentless, often spilling over into late nights and early mornings. The pressure to perform and the constant juggling of responsibilities affected her mental and emotional well-being. To cope with the stress, Sarah found herself turning to food. Late-night binge-eating sessions became a routine, a way to unwind after a grueling day. She would reach for anything that offered quick comfort—chocolate, chips, ice cream—all the while knowing this wasn't a healthy way to deal with her emotions.

The aftermath of these binge sessions was always the same. Sarah would wake up feeling guilty and ashamed, her stomach heavy and her mind clouded with regret. She would promise herself that it wouldn't happen again, but the cycle continued. The weight started to pile on, and she began experiencing digestive issues that only added to her stress. It was a vicious loop that seemed impossible to break. The impact on her physical health was undeniable, but the emotional burden was even more overwhelming. She felt trapped in a cycle of self-criticism and despair, unable to see a way out.

The turning point in Sarah's journey came during a routine check-up. Her doctor expressed concern about her weight gain and the digestive problems she was experiencing. It was a wake-up call that made her realize how much her emotional eating affected her overall health. Around the same time, a close friend noticed Sarah's struggles and initiated a heartfelt conversation. This friend shared her own experiences with emotional eating and encouraged Sarah to seek help. A moment of vulnerability and connection sparked a desire for change in Sarah.

Determined to reclaim her health and well-being, Sarah sought help from a therapist specializing in cognitive-behavioral therapy (CBT). Through treatment, she began to understand the underlying emotions driving her eating habits. She learned to identify her triggers and develop healthier ways to cope with stress and anxiety. The therapist introduced her to mindful eating, which encourages being fully present during meals and listening to the body's hunger and satiety cues. Sarah started journaling her thoughts and feelings, which helped her gain insights into her emotional patterns and eating behaviors.

Building a support network was another crucial step in Sarah's recovery. She confided in her close friends and family, sharing her struggles and asking for their support. This openness fostered a sense of accountability and encouragement that bolstered her efforts. Her friends would check in on her progress, and her family started to adopt healthier eating habits, creating a supportive environment that made it easier for Sarah to stay on track.

Sarah's journey wasn't without its challenges. Sometimes, she slipped back into old habits, but she learned to approach these moments with self-compassion rather than self-criticism. Each setback became an opportunity for growth, a chance to reinforce her commitment to healthier coping mechanisms. Over time, Sarah noticed significant improvements in her physical health. Her digestive issues began to resolve, and she started to lose weight healthily and sustainably. More importantly, she felt a sense of emotional freedom and empowerment that she hadn't experienced in years.

Sarah's story is a testament to the power of awareness, support, and self-compassion in overcoming emotional eating. It reminds us that change is possible, even when the path seems daunting. By seeking help, practicing mindfulness, and building a supportive network, Sarah transformed her relationship with food and, ultimately, her life.

Journaling Exercise

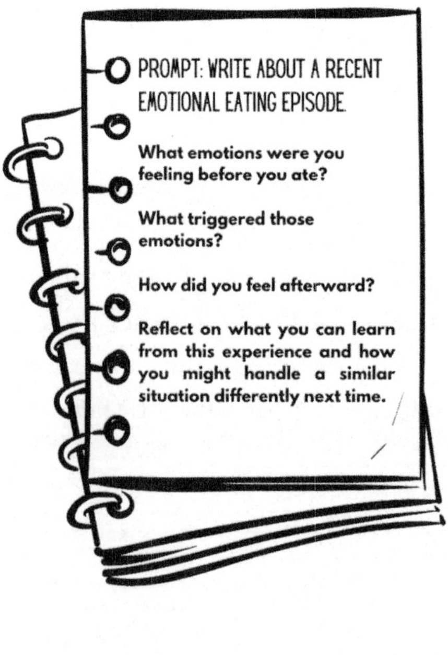

FINDING BALANCE: JOE'S STORY OF RECOVERY

Meet Joe, a driven entrepreneur who built his own tech startup from the ground up. His days were filled with back-to-back meetings, client presentations, and countless emails. The pressure to keep his business afloat and thriving was immense, leaving little room for anything else. Joe often worked late into the night, his desk littered with fast food wrappers and empty soda cans. The fast-paced nature of his career made maintaining a work-life balance almost impossible. Between the endless deadlines and the constant need to perform, Mark started to rely on food as a quick fix for his stress and exhaustion.

Joe's emotional eating manifested during those late-night work sessions. With the clock ticking past midnight and his to-do list still looming large, he would turn to fast food and sugary snacks. They were convenient and provided a temporary sense of relief. But this habit took a toll on his energy levels and productivity. The sugar highs were followed by inevitable crashes, leaving him more drained and less focused. His diet was wreaking havoc on his body, and he found himself in a never-ending cycle of fatigue and poor eating choices. Emotional eating became a way to cope with the relentless stress and pressure of his job, but it only compounded his problems.

The turning point for Joe came when he experienced a health scare that jolted him into reality. One evening, he felt a sharp pain in his chest and shortness of breath. A trip to the emergency room revealed that his blood pressure was alarmingly high, and his cholesterol levels were through the roof. The doctor warned him that if he didn't make significant lifestyle changes, he was at serious risk for heart disease. This wake-up call made Joe realize the dire consequences of his lifestyle. Around the same time, his partner expressed concern about his health and encouraged him to seek a healthier lifestyle. This combination of factors was a powerful motivator for Joe to change his habits.

Determined to turn his life around, Joe hired a nutrition coach. Together, they worked on planning balanced meals that were both nutritious and satisfying. The coach helped him understand the importance of fueling his body with nutrients and providing practical tips for healthier food choices. Joe started incorporating more fruits, vegetables, and whole grains into his diet, gradually phasing out the fast food and sugary snacks that had become his go-to. This shift improved his physical health and gave him more sustained energy throughout the day.

In addition to changing his diet, Joe recognized the need for regular physical activity. He began incorporating exercise into his daily routine, starting with simple activities like walking and gradually progressing to more intensive workouts. Exercise became a way for him to release stress and boost his mood. The endorphins from physical activity helped counterbalance the stress hormones that had been contributing to his emotional eating. Mark found that regular exercise improved his physical fitness and enhanced his mental clarity and focus, making him more productive at work.

Mindfulness and stress management techniques played a crucial role in Joe's recovery. He started practicing mindfulness meditation, which helped him become more aware of his thoughts and emotions without judgment. This practice allowed him to recognize when he was feeling stressed or overwhelmed and to address those feelings in healthier ways. He also learned deep breathing exercises and progressive muscle relaxation, which he used to calm his mind and body during stressful moments. These techniques provided him with alternative coping mechanisms, reducing his reliance on food for comfort.

Joe's journey was not without its challenges. He struggled to maintain his new habits, especially during particularly stressful periods at work. However, he learned to approach these setbacks with self-compassion and perseverance. Each time he faced a challenge, he reminded himself of his progress and the reasons behind his commitment to a healthier lifestyle. Over time, Joe noticed significant improvements in his physical health, including lower blood pressure and cholesterol levels. His energy levels stabilized, and he felt more in control of his eating habits.

Joe's story is a powerful example of how awareness, support, and mindfulness can transform one's relationship with food and well-being. By seeking professional help, embracing physical activity, and adopting mindfulness techniques, Joe found balance and overcame the grip of emotional eating. His experience inspires anyone facing similar struggles, showing that positive change is possible with dedication and the proper support.

THE POWER OF SUPPORT: MIA'S PATH TO HEALING

Mia was a stay-at-home mom, a role she loved but found incredibly isolating. Her days were filled with the endless tasks of parenting—cooking meals, cleaning up messes, and managing tantrums. Despite being surrounded by her family, Mia often felt a deep sense of loneliness. Her husband worked long hours, and her friends were busy with their own lives. The constant demands of her children left her with little time for herself, and she frequently found herself alone in the house, craving comfort.

Mia's emotional eating began as a way to fill the void she felt during those lonely moments at home. Whenever her kids were napping or playing quietly, she wandered into the kitchen, looking for something to snack on. A cookie here, a handful of chips there

—it didn't seem like much then, but it added up. Food became her solace, a way to distract herself from the isolation and stress of parenting. The more she turned to food, the more she began to rely on it to cope with her emotions. Her self-esteem took a hit, and she started to feel trapped in a cycle of emotional eating and self-criticism.

The stress of parenting only amplified her struggles. The constant pressure to be the perfect mom weighed heavily on her. She felt like she had to maintain a flawless home, provide nutritious meals, and be emotionally available for her children. This unrealistic standard left her feeling inadequate and stressed. Whenever she felt overwhelmed, she turned to food for comfort. The short-lived relief it provided was quickly replaced by guilt and shame, further eroding her self-esteem and body image. Mia began to notice the physical toll it was taking on her body. She gained weight and felt sluggish, adding to her feelings of inadequacy.

The turning point came during a playgroup session with other moms. One of the mothers noticed Mia's distress and struck up a conversation. As they talked, Mia found herself opening up about her struggles with loneliness and emotional eating. The other mom shared her experiences and mentioned a local support group for moms with similar issues. This heartfelt discussion was a revelation for Mia. She realized she wasn't alone, and that seeking support was not a sign of weakness but a step towards healing.

Determined to make a change, Mia decided to join the support group. The group met weekly, providing a safe space for moms to share their experiences and encourage each other. Emily found solace in the camaraderie and understanding of other women going through similar struggles. The group sessions became a lifeline, giving her the emotional support she had lacked. She also started to build a routine that included self-care and social activities. Emily began setting aside time each day for activities she enjoyed, like reading, gardening, and taking short walks. These moments of self-care helped her reconnect with herself and provided a healthy outlet for her emotions.

Seeking professional help was another crucial step in Mia's path to recovery. She reached out to a counselor who specialized in parenting-related emotional issues. Through therapy, Mia explored the underlying emotions driving her eating habits. She learned to identify her triggers and develop healthier ways to cope with stress and loneliness. The counselor introduced her to mindfulness techniques, which helped her become more aware of her emotional state and make more conscious choices about her eating. Mia started journaling her thoughts and feelings, which provided valuable insights into her emotional patterns and helped her track her progress.

Mia's journey was also not without its challenges. There were days when she felt overwhelmed and tempted to revert to old habits. However, she learned to approach these moments with self-compassion rather than self-criticism. Each setback became an opportunity for growth, reinforcing her commitment to healthier coping mechanisms. Over time, Emily noticed significant improvements in her self-esteem and body image. She felt more in control of her eating habits and experienced a renewed sense of confidence. The support group, her new routine, and therapy provided a strong foundation for lasting change.

Mia's story is a testament to the power of support and self-care in overcoming emotional eating. It highlights the importance of seeking help, building a supportive network, and making time for oneself. Through these efforts, Emily transformed her relationship with food. She found a healthier, more balanced way to navigate parenting challenges.

EMBRACING SELF-LOVE: TINA'S TRANSFORMATION

Tina's life has always revolved around the fashion industry, where beauty standards are rigid and unforgiving. From a young age, Tina was captivated by the allure of fashion magazines and runway shows. However, this fascination came with its own set of challenges. She struggled with body image and self-esteem, often feeling like she never quite measured up to the models she admired. Tina's history with dieting began in her teenage years, influenced by the constant pressure to look a certain way. She tried every diet imaginable, from low carb to juice cleanses, but nothing seemed to bring lasting satisfaction. Instead, she found herself caught in a cycle of yo-yo dieting and binge eating, her weight fluctuating wildly as she swung from one extreme to the other.

Working in the fashion industry only amplified these struggles. Surrounded by thin, glamorous colleagues and models, Tina felt immense pressure to conform to the industry's beauty standards. The constant scrutiny and comparison took a toll on her mental health. Emotional eating became her way of coping with feelings of inadequacy. After a long day at work, she would come home and binge on whatever comfort food she could find—ice cream, pizza, chips. These moments provided temporary relief but were quickly followed by intense guilt and self-loathing. The emotional eating cycles exacerbated her anxiety and depression, creating a vicious loop that seemed impossible to escape.

The turning point for Tina came when she attended a body positivity workshop on a friend's recommendation. The workshop was a revelation. For the first time, she heard voices that challenged the narrow beauty standards she had internalized for so long. The experience was eye-opening and deeply moving. Here, Tina had an empowering conversation with a body-positive influencer who shared her struggles with body image and self-acceptance. This conversation struck a chord with Tina, igniting a desire to change her approach to her body and her eating habits.

Determined to embrace self-love and break free from the cycle of emotional eating, Tina began practicing self-compassion. She started by incorporating body-positive affirmations into her daily routine. Each morning, she would look in the mirror and speak words of kindness and acceptance to herself. This practice helped shift her mindset from one of self-criticism to one of self-love. Tina also explored activities that promoted self-acceptance. She joined a body-positive yoga class, focusing on how the body felt rather than how it looked. These classes became a sanctuary for her, where she could reconnect with her body in a nurturing and supportive environment.

Building a community of like-minded individuals was another crucial step in her transformation. Tina joined online forums and social media groups dedicated to body positivity and self-love. These communities provided a sense of belonging and encouragement that she had been missing. She found inspiration in the stories of others on similar paths, reinforcing her commitment to her own healing. The support from these communities helped Tina realize that she was not alone in her struggles and that change was possible.

As Tina continued on this path of self-discovery, she noticed significant improvements in her mental health. Her anxiety and depression began to lift, and she felt a renewed sense of confidence and well-being. The binge eating episodes became less frequent as she developed healthier ways to cope with her emotions. Tina's relationship with food transformed; it was no longer a source of guilt and shame but one of nourishment and enjoyment. She learned to listen to her body's hunger and satiety cues, practicing mindful eating and savoring each bite.

Tina's journey of embracing self-love and overcoming emotional eating has been a testament to the power of self-compassion, community, and positive affirmations. Her story reminds us that it is possible to break free from the confines of societal beauty standards and find true acceptance within oneself.

FROM STRUGGLE TO STRENGTH: ALEX'S INSPIRING TALE

Meet Alex, a competitive athlete whose life revolved around rigorous training, intense competitions, and the constant pressure to perform at his best. From a young age, Alex was driven by the thrill of competition and the desire to excel in his sport. He dedicated countless hours to training, pushing his body to its limits in pursuit of victory. But beneath the surface, the pressure to succeed took a toll on his relationship with food. Performance pressures and the need to maintain a specific weight and physique led Alex down a path of emotional eating struggles that deeply affected both his athletic performance and mental health.

The demands of being a top athlete created a high-stress environment for Alex. Every competition felt like a test of his worth, and the fear of failure loomed large. After a tough loss or a challenging training session, he would turn to food for comfort. Emotional eating became a way to cope with the intense pressure and the fear of not measuring up. Alex's binge eating episodes often followed competition losses, where he would consume large quantities of food to numb the disappointment and frustration. These episodes provided temporary relief but were always followed by guilt and self-reproach.

The impact on his athletic performance was significant. The physical discomfort and lethargy from overeating hindered his training, making it harder for him to maintain the high level of performance expected of him. His mental health also suffered. The constant cycle of binge eating, and self-criticism eroded his confidence and left him feeling trapped in a loop of unhealthy behaviors. Alex found it increasingly difficult to separate his self-worth from his performance, and food became a refuge and a source of shame.

The turning point for Alex came during a candid conversation with his coach. Recognizing the signs of distress, his coach gently brought up the topic of mental health. This open dialogue was a crucial moment for Alex. He realized that his struggles were not just about food but also about the immense pressure he was under. His coach encouraged him to attend a workshop on emotional resilience designed for athletes. The workshop provided Alex with new perspectives and tools to manage stress and emotions in healthier ways.

Determined to address the underlying issues, Alex began working with a sports psychologist. Through therapy, he explored the deep-seated emotions driving his eating habits and learned to identify his triggers. The psychologist introduced him to mindfulness and stress reduction techniques, which became vital to his recovery. Alex started practicing mindfulness meditation, which helped him become more aware of his thoughts and feelings without judgment. This practice allowed him to recognize when he felt overwhelmed and address those emotions more effectively.

Implementing these techniques, Alex began to foster a balanced approach to training and self-care. He learned the importance of listening to his body and giving it the rest and nourishment it needed. Instead of pushing himself to the brink, he started incorporating rest days and recovery activities into his training regimen. This balanced approach not only improved his physical health but also enhanced his mental well-being. Alex found that when he treated his body with kindness and respect, his performance improved, and he felt more in control of his eating habits.

Building a support network was another crucial step in Alex's path to strength. He confided in his teammates and close friends, sharing his struggles and seeking their support. This openness fostered a sense of accountability and encouragement that bolstered his efforts. His teammates became a source of motivation, reminding him to prioritize his well-being and to approach setbacks with resilience. The support network created an environment where Alex felt understood and valued, which played a significant role in his recovery.

Alex's story is a powerful reminder that it is possible to find strength and resilience even in the face of immense pressure. By seeking professional help, practicing mindfulness, and building a supportive network, Alex transformed his relationship with food and his approach to his sport. His journey illustrates that true strength comes from recognizing and addressing our vulnerabilities and that we can overcome even the most challenging struggles with the right tools and support.

CHAPTER 9

PRACTICAL TOOLS AND TECHNIQUES

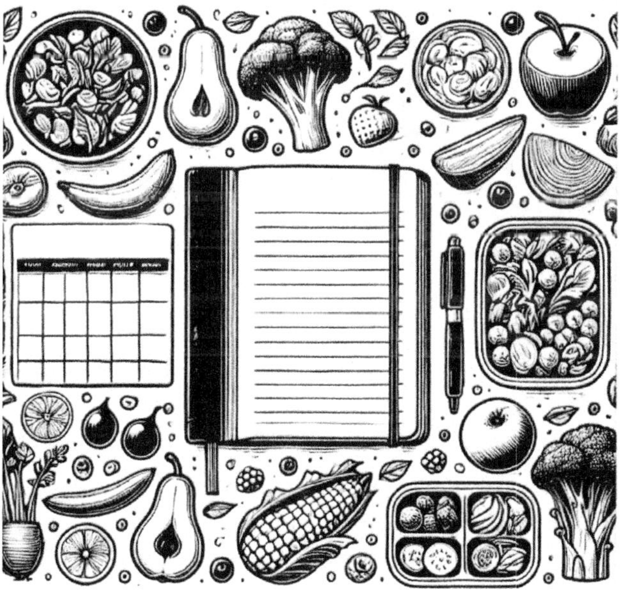

FOOD DIARIES: TRACKING YOUR EATING HABITS

The concept of keeping a food diary is simple yet profound. You gain valuable insights into your eating habits by writing down what you eat and when you eat it. But a food diary is more than just a list of meals and snacks. It's a tool for tracking your emotional state and the context in which you eat. Doing this allows you to identify patterns and triggers that lead to emotional eating. For instance, you might notice that you reach for sugary snacks when stressed at work or that you overeat during social gatherings. This awareness is the first step toward change.

Accurately and consistently recording your food intake can seem challenging, but it doesn't have to be. The key is to choose a format that works best for you. Some people prefer the simplicity of pen and paper. In contrast, others might opt for digital apps that offer added features like reminders and analysis. Whichever method you choose, the important thing is to be honest and detailed in your entries. Note not just what you eat but also how you're feeling and what's happening around you at the time.

Here's a detailed example to illustrate what a food diary entry might look like: "10 AM: Ate a granola bar; felt stressed about a work deadline." This entry not only records the food but also provides context and emotion, making it easier to spot patterns later. Another example could be, "7 PM: Had pasta for dinner; felt relaxed and happy." These details are crucial for understanding the emotional backdrop of your eating habits.

When you analyze your food diary, look for common emotional triggers. You may find specific emotions consistently lead to overeating. For instance, noticing that you often eat when bored is a valuable insight. Pay attention to time-of-day patterns as well. Are you more likely to snack late at night or during mid-afternoon slumps? Recognizing these patterns can help you anticipate and manage your emotional eating.

Specific foods frequently consumed during emotional eating episodes can also provide clues. For example, seeing that you always reach for chocolate when you're feeling down is a trigger to explore further. Understanding these details helps you develop strategies for managing emotional eating, such as finding healthier alternatives or directly addressing underlying emotions.

Daily Food Diary Template

To get started, here's a simple template you can use for your food diary:

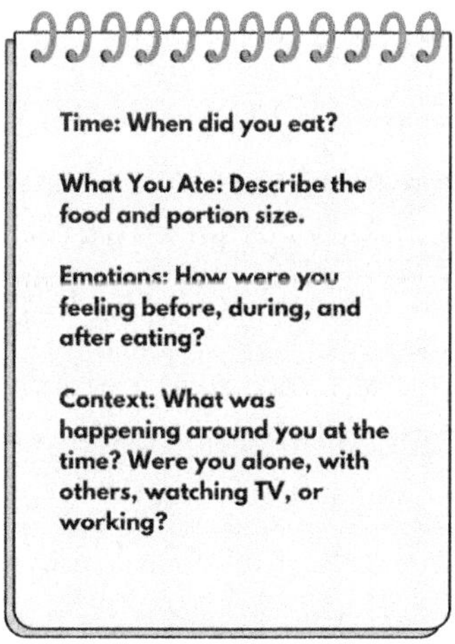

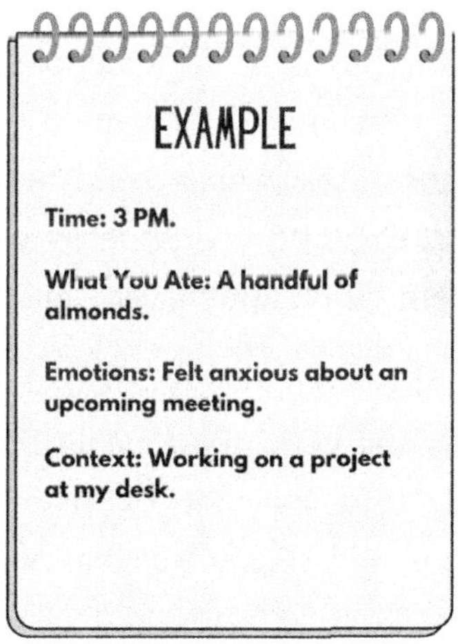

By consistently using this template, you'll gather valuable data over time, making it easier to spot patterns and triggers. The more detailed you are, the better. Reflecting on these entries can offer profound insights into your relationship with food and emotions, paving the way for healthier habits.

MINDFUL MEAL PLANNING: CREATING A BALANCED MENU

Meal planning can be a game-changer when it comes to combating emotional eating. Planning meals in advance helps reduce impulsive eating decisions, often driven by emotions rather than genuine hunger. By knowing what you'll eat throughout the day, you can avoid those moments when you reach for unhealthy snacks or fast food simply because you didn't have a plan. This foresight ensures that your diet remains balanced, providing all the nutrients your body needs to function optimally.

Mindful meal planning starts with incorporating a variety of food groups into your daily meals. This approach ensures nutritional balance and keeps your meals exciting and satisfying. Consider including fruits, vegetables, whole grains, proteins, and healthy fats in your diet. For example, a breakfast of oatmeal topped with fresh berries and a sprinkle of nuts provides fiber, vitamins, and healthy fats. Lunch could be a quinoa salad with mixed greens, chickpeas, and a drizzle of olive oil, offering a good balance of protein, fiber, and healthy fats.

Planning snacks and meals throughout the day is as essential as preparing your main meals. Snacks can help maintain your energy levels and prevent overeating at mealtime. Consider healthy options like a handful of almonds, fruit, or yogurt with honey and seeds. Portion sizes and hunger levels should guide your meal planning. Be mindful of how much you're eating and whether it aligns with your hunger cues. Smaller plates can help control portions, and attention to your body's signals can prevent overeating. Sample meal plans can serve as a helpful guide.

- For those who follow a vegetarian diet, a day might look like this: Breakfast with a smoothie made from spinach, banana, and almond milk; a lunch of lentil soup with a side of whole grain bread; a snack of hummus with carrot sticks; and a dinner of vegetable stir-fry with tofu over brown rice.
- For omnivores, a balanced day could include scrambled eggs with veggies for breakfast, a chicken salad for lunch, a snack of Greek yogurt with berries, and grilled salmon with quinoa and roasted vegetables for dinner.
- Gluten-free individuals might enjoy an avocado toast made with gluten-free bread for breakfast, a quinoa and black bean salad for lunch, an apple with almond butter for a snack, and a dinner of grilled chicken with sweet potatoes and steamed broccoli.

Flexibility is vital in mindful meal planning. Life is unpredictable, and your meal plans should be adaptable. If a meeting runs late or you're invited out for an impromptu dinner, adjusting your plans is okay. Allow yourself occasional indulgences without guilt. The goal is balance, not perfection. Enjoy a piece of chocolate cake mindfully and without remorse if you crave it. This approach helps prevent feelings of deprivation.

Adapting to changing schedules is another crucial aspect. If you have a busy week ahead, plan simple and quick meals requiring minimal preparation. Batch cooking on weekends can save time during the week, providing healthy meals even on your busiest days. Preparing a big pot of soup or a tray of roasted vegetables used in various weekly meals can be a lifesaver.

Incorporating these strategies into your routine can make a significant difference in managing emotional eating. By planning your meals mindfully, you create a structure that supports healthy eating habits and reduces the likelihood of making impulsive food choices driven by emotions.

HEALTHY SNACKING: ALTERNATIVES TO EMOTIONAL EATING

Healthy snacks play an important role in maintaining a balanced diet. They can provide sustained energy throughout the day, helping you stay focused and productive. They act as bridges between meals, ensuring you don't arrive at your next meal feeling ravenous and prone to overeating.

Choosing the right snacks can make all the difference. Whole foods are your best bet over-processed options. Think of fruits, vegetables, nuts, and seeds. These foods are packed with nutrients and are free from added sugars and unhealthy fats. Balancing macronutrients in your snacks is also important. Aim for a mix of protein, carbs, and fats to keep you full and satisfied. For example, a handful of almonds (protein and fat) paired with an apple (carbs) can provide a well-rounded snack that keeps you energized. There are plenty of easy-to-prepare, nutritious snack options to consider.

- Greek yogurt with berries offers a delightful combination of protein and antioxidants. Hummus with carrot sticks provides fiber and healthy fats, making it a filling choice.
- Apple slices with almond butter are a fantastic mix of crunch and creaminess, offering carbohydrates and protein.
- Mixed nuts and seeds are another excellent option. They are rich in healthy fats and protein and are perfect for a quick, satisfying bite.

To make snacking a mindful practice, start by eating slowly and savoring each bite. This approach helps you appreciate the flavors and textures of your food, enhancing the eating experience. Pay attention to your hunger and fullness cues. Before reaching for a snack, ask yourself if you're truly hungry or eating out of habit or emotion. If you're genuinely hungry, enjoy your snack mindfully, stopping when satisfied. Avoid distractions while snacking. Eating in front of the TV or while working can lead to mindless munching, where you might eat more than you intended. Instead, sit down and focus on your snack for a few moments.

SNACK PREPARATION CHECKLIST

To make healthy snacking easier, here's a simple checklist you can follow:

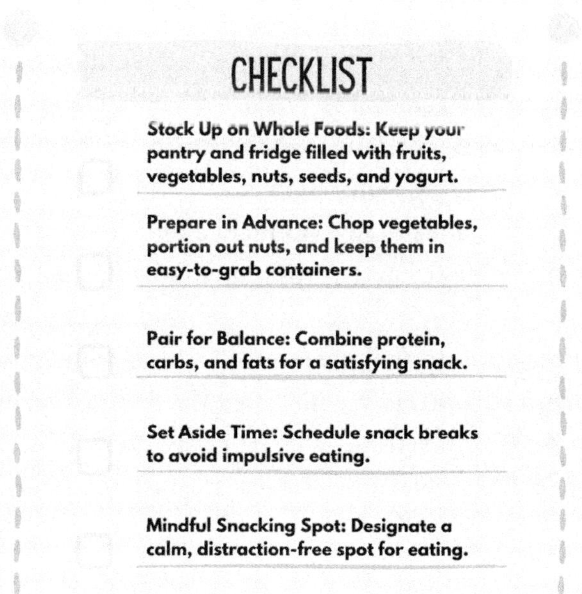
CHECKLIST
Stock Up on Whole Foods: Keep your pantry and fridge filled with fruits, vegetables, nuts, seeds, and yogurt.
Prepare in Advance: Chop vegetables, portion out nuts, and keep them in easy-to-grab containers.
Pair for Balance: Combine protein, carbs, and fats for a satisfying snack.
Set Aside Time: Schedule snack breaks to avoid impulsive eating.
Mindful Snacking Spot: Designate a calm, distraction-free spot for eating.

By following this checklist, you'll find it easier to choose healthy snacks and enjoy them mindfully. This approach can help prevent emotional eating and steady your energy levels throughout the day.

Healthy snacking isn't about deprivation or rigid rules; it's about making choices that nourish your body and mind. By prioritizing whole foods and balancing macronutrients, you can enjoy snacks that keep you full and satisfied. Mindful practices enhance the experience, ensuring that you're not just eating to fill a void but genuinely enjoying the nourishment. Remember, the goal is to create a sustainable habit that supports your overall well-being, making it easier to manage emotional eating and maintain a balanced diet.

SETTING REALISTIC GOALS: SMALL STEPS TO BIG CHANGES

Setting realistic goals is a cornerstone of overcoming emotional eating. When you set achievable goals, you create a pathway to long-term success. Imagine the satisfaction of reaching a small milestone, like journaling your food intake three times a week. Each small victory builds your confidence and motivates you to keep going. On the other hand, setting unattainable goals can lead to discouragement and self-criticism, which can trigger emotional eating. It's about finding that sweet spot where your goals challenge you but are still within reach. Using the SMART criteria can be incredibly helpful in setting realistic goals. SMART stands for Specific, Measurable, Achievable, Relevant, and Time-bound.

- Specific goals are clear and precise, leaving no room for ambiguity. For example, instead of saying, "I want to eat healthier," you could say, "I will include a serving of vegetables in every meal this week."
- Measurable goals allow you to track your progress. If you want to practice mindful eating, you might decide to do it during dinner every night.
- Achievable goals are realistic and within your capabilities. Setting a goal to run a marathon next month if you've never run before is likely setting yourself up for failure. Instead, aim for smaller steps, like jogging for 20 minutes thrice weekly.
- Relevant goals align with your broader objectives and values. If your primary aim is to overcome emotional eating, setting a goal to meditate daily can be more appropriate than a goal unrelated to your eating habits.
- Finally, Time-bound goals have a deadline, which keeps you focused and motivated. Saying, "I will try one new healthy snack this week," gives you a clear timeframe to work within.

Breaking larger goals into smaller steps makes them manageable. If your ultimate goal is to develop a healthier relationship with food, start with smaller steps, like identifying one emotional eating trigger and finding a new way to cope. Each small step you take is a building block toward your larger goal. For instance, instead of aiming to eliminate all emotional eating immediately, you might start by practicing mindful eating at one meal each day. As you become more comfortable with this practice, you can gradually expand it to other meals. This incremental approach helps you build confidence and provides a sense of accomplishment.

Here are some realistic goals related to emotional eating: "I will journal my food intake three times this week." This goal is specific, measurable, achievable, relevant, and time bound. Another example is, "I will practice mindful eating at dinner every night this week." This goal focuses on a specific meal, making it manageable and easy to track. Lastly, "I will try one new healthy snack this week" is a simple yet effective goal that encourages you to explore nutritious options without overwhelming you.

Tracking your progress is crucial for staying motivated and making adjustments as needed. Keeping a goal-tracking journal can help you monitor your achievements and reflect on your challenges. Write down your goals and note your progress regularly. Celebrate milestones and accomplishments, no matter how small they may seem. Did you manage to practice mindful eating every night this week? Give yourself a pat on the back. Recognizing and celebrating your successes boosts your confidence and keeps you motivated.

Reflecting on challenges is equally important. If you didn't meet a goal, take a moment to understand why. Were there unexpected obstacles? Did you set a goal that was too ambitious? Use these reflections to adjust your goals and strategies. For instance, if you find journaling your daily food intake challenging, try reducing the frequency to three times a week. The key is to be flexible and kind to yourself. Adjust your goals based on your experiences and learnings. This iterative process helps you find what works best for you and ensures your goals remain realistic and achievable.

Goal-Tracking Exercise

To help you track your progress and stay motivated, try this simple exercise:

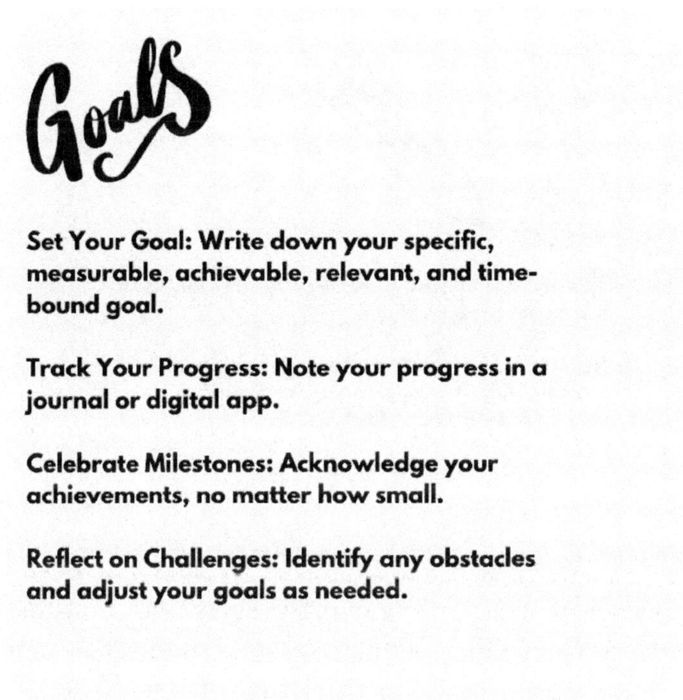

EXAMPLE

Goal: Practice mindful eating at dinner every night this week.

Progress:
Mon: ✓
Tue: ✓
Wed: ✗
Thu: ✓
Fri: ✓
Sat: ✗
Sun: ✓

Milestone: Successfully practiced mindful eating for six out of seven nights.

Reflection: I missed Wednesday due to a late meeting. Adjusted by planning for a quick, mindful meal on busy days.

Setting realistic goals and tracking progress can transform your approach to overcoming emotional eating. Each small step builds momentum, leading to significant, lasting changes. Remember, the journey to a healthier relationship with food is not a sprint but a series of small, consistent steps.

CREATING A SUPPORTIVE ENVIRONMENT: HOME AND WORK

Creating a supportive environment is crucial for combating emotional eating. Your surroundings can help you make healthier choices or tempt you into old habits. Reducing exposure to triggers and encouraging healthy behaviors at home and work can make a significant difference. Think of your environment as your ally in this journey. By making small but impactful changes, you can create spaces that support your goals and make it easier to stick to healthier habits.

At home, start by stocking your pantry with healthy options. Fill your shelves with whole foods like fruits, vegetables, nuts, and whole grains. When healthy choices are readily available, you're more likely to reach for them. Conversely, removing or limiting access to trigger foods can reduce temptation. If you know that chips and cookies are your go-to comfort foods, keep them out of sight, or better yet, don't buy them. Setting up a designated mindful eating space can also be beneficial. Choose a calm, clutter-free area where you can eat without distractions. This space should be free from screens and distractions, allowing you to focus on your meal and savor each bite.

The challenges can be different in the work environment but just as significant. Bringing healthy snacks and meals from home can help you avoid the pitfalls of the office snack drawer or vending machines. Prepare your snacks and meals the night before to ensure you have nutritious options. Taking mindful breaks to eat is another important strategy. Eating lunch at your desk while working is easy, but this often leads to mindless eating. Instead, step away from your workspace to a quiet area to focus on your meal. This helps you eat more mindfully and gives you a mental break, which can improve your overall productivity.

Creating a supportive environment is about making your spaces work for you. This might mean decluttering your kitchen, organizing your pantry, or creating a peaceful eating nook at home. It could involve bringing your own meals, finding a quiet place to eat, or even talking to your colleagues about healthier snack options in the office. These changes may seem small but can significantly impact your eating habits and overall well-being.

Remember, the goal is to make healthy choices as easy and automatic as possible. By surrounding yourself with healthy options and creating spaces that encourage mindful eating, you set yourself up for success. You'll find it easier to resist emotional eating triggers and stay on track with your goals. Each small change in your environment brings you closer to a healthier, more balanced relationship with food.

As you continue to create these supportive environments, you'll notice that making healthier choices becomes more natural. You'll feel more in control of your eating habits and less reliant on food for emotional comfort. This proactive approach helps you manage emotional eating and fosters a sense of empowerment and well-being. Taking charge of your surroundings creates a foundation for lasting change and a healthier, happier life.

CHAPTER 10

SUSTAINABLE CHANGE AND LONG-TERM SUCCESS

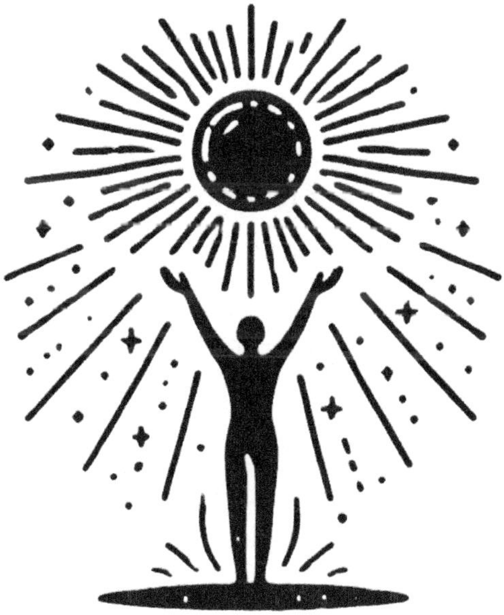

Visualize waking up on a Saturday morning, feeling refreshed and ready to face the day. You have your breakfast planned, your workout gear is laid out, and you know exactly what you'll do to care for yourself. This sense of readiness doesn't come overnight; it results from building consistent habits that support your well-being. Sustainable change and long-term success in overcoming emotional eating hinge on the consistency of these healthy habits. Maintaining this consistency is essential for lasting improvements in your relationship with food and overall well-being.

MAINTAINING PROGRESS: STRATEGIES FOR LONG-TERM SUCCESS

Consistency is the backbone of sustainable change. When you maintain healthy habits regularly, they become second nature, integrated seamlessly into your daily routine. One way to build this consistency is by creating daily routines that revolve around healthy eating and self-care. For instance, setting a specific time for meals, incorporating regular physical activity, and ensuring you have moments of relaxation and mindfulness throughout your day can make a significant difference. These routines create a structure that makes it easier to stick to healthy habits, even when life gets hectic.

Setting reminders for mindfulness practices can also help you stay consistent. Use your phone or a journal to remind yourself to take deep breaths, meditate, or check in with your emotions before reaching for a snack. These small practices can accumulate over time, helping you build a stronger foundation for managing emotional eating. Another practical tip is to keep a regular food and emotion journal. Documenting what you eat and how you feel can provide insights into your eating patterns and emotional triggers. By reviewing your journal regularly, you can identify areas for improvement and celebrate your progress.

Scheduling regular check-ins with a support network or therapist is another effective strategy for staying on track. These check-ins provide accountability and allow you to discuss any challenges you face. Whether it's a weekly call with a friend or a monthly session with a therapist, these conversations can offer support and encouragement, helping you stay committed to your goals. Planning ahead for challenging situations, such as holidays or periods of high stress, is also crucial. Anticipate potential triggers and develop strategies to manage them. For example, if you know that holidays are challenging, plan healthy meals and snacks in advance and set boundaries around food-related activities.

Adaptability plays a significant role in maintaining progress. Life is dynamic, and your strategies must evolve with changing circumstances. Adapting meal plans to new routines or dietary needs ensures that you continue to nourish your body in a way that supports your well-being. For instance, if you start a new job with different hours, adjust your meal and snack times to fit your new schedule. Similarly, being flexible with exercise routines is important. If you're experiencing physical limitations or a busy period, modify your workouts to match your current capabilities. The key is to remain active and engaged with your health, even if the specifics of your routine change.

Maintaining progress isn't about perfection; it's about consistency and adaptability. You can achieve long-term success by building daily routines around healthy eating and self-care, setting reminders for mindfulness practices, and staying flexible with your strategies. It's also important to keep a food and emotion journal, schedule regular check-ins with a support network, and plan ahead for challenging situations.

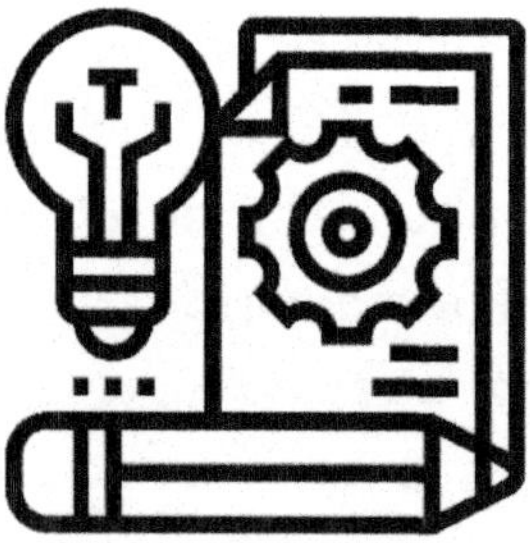

ADAPTABILITY CHECKLIST

Assess your current routine and identify and changes in your schedule or lifestyle.

Adjust meal plans to fit new routines or dietary needs.

Modify exercise routines based on physical capabilities or time constraints.

Plan ahead for challenging situations and develop strategies to manage triggers.

Use reminders and journaling to stay consistent with mindfulness practices.

Schedule regular check-ins with a support network or therapist.

CELEBRATING MILESTONES: ACKNOWLEDGING YOUR ACHIEVEMENTS

Imagine you've been working hard to develop healthier eating habits and manage your emotional eating triggers. One day, you realize it's been six months since you last turned to food for comfort. This is a milestone worth celebrating! Recognizing and celebrating your achievements is crucial for maintaining motivation and boosting self-esteem. When you acknowledge your progress, you reinforce positive behavior and build confidence in your ability to make lasting changes. Each milestone, no matter how small, is a testament to your effort and resilience.

Reinforcing positive behavior through celebration creates a positive feedback loop. When you celebrate your achievements, you message yourself that your efforts are worthwhile and meaningful. This reinforcement can make staying committed to your goals more accessible, even when faced with challenges. Building confidence and self-efficacy is another important aspect of celebrating milestones. When you see tangible evidence of your progress, you start to believe in your ability to overcome obstacles and achieve your goals. This growing sense of self-efficacy can empower you to take on new challenges and strive for improvement.

There are many creative and meaningful ways to celebrate your achievements. Treating yourself to a non-food-related reward can be incredibly satisfying and fulfilling. For example, you might indulge in a spa day, buy a new book you've wanted to read, or take a day trip to a place you've always wanted to visit. These rewards acknowledge your hard work and provide an opportunity for relaxation and enjoyment, reinforcing the positive changes you've made. Sharing your successes with a supportive community or loved ones can also be a powerful way to celebrate. When you share your achievements, you invite others to join your celebration and provide encouragement and support. This sense of community can strengthen your resolve and make your accomplishments feel even more meaningful.

Self-reflection plays a crucial role in celebrating milestones. Taking the time to reflect on your journey and accomplishments can help you appreciate your progress and gain insights into what has worked well for you. Journaling about your personal growth and successes can be a valuable tool for reflection. Write about the challenges you've faced, the strategies you've used, and the progress you've made. This process can help you recognize patterns, identify strengths, and plan for future growth. Creating a visual representation of your progress, such as a vision board, can also be a powerful way to celebrate and reflect. A vision board allows you to visually capture your goals, achievements, and aspirations, constantly reminding you of your progress and motivation.

CELEBRATING YOUR MILESTONES

Take a moment to reflect on your recent achievements and progress. Write down at least three milestones you've reached in your journey to manage emotional eating and build healthier habits.

Consider how you can celebrate these milestones meaningfully and rewardingly. Consider non-food-related rewards that bring you joy and fulfillment.

Write a short journal entry about each milestone, describing the challenges you faced, the strategies you used, and the progress you made. Reflect on how these achievements have impacted your well-being and self-esteem.

Create a visual representation of your progress, such as a vision board. Include images, quotes, and symbols that represent your goals and achievements. Place this visual reminder somewhere you can see it daily to keep you motivated and inspired.

Celebrating milestones is not just about recognizing your achievements; it's about reinforcing positive behavior, building confidence, and nurturing self-efficacy. By treating yourself to non-food-related rewards and sharing your successes with a supportive community, you acknowledge the hard work and dedication you've invested in your well-being. Self-reflection through journaling and creating visual representations of your progress can deepen your appreciation for your journey and provide ongoing motivation.

CONTINUOUS GROWTH: EMBRACING A LIFELONG JOURNEY

Overcoming emotional eating is a marathon, not a sprint. It's an ongoing process. Embracing a lifelong growth mindset means viewing each step, each stumble, and each stride forward as part of your ongoing development. Setbacks aren't failures; they're opportunities to learn and grow. Each challenge you face can teach you something new about yourself and your relationship with food.

Continuous self-improvement is about committing to your personal development every single day. This commitment involves staying curious and open to learning. Reading books, articles, and research on emotional eating and related topics can expand your understanding and provide new insights. Attending workshops, seminars, or support groups offers a chance to connect with others who share similar struggles and goals. These interactions can provide fresh perspectives and practical strategies to incorporate into your routine. Engaging with a community of like-minded individuals helps reinforce your commitment to growth and keeps you motivated.

Setting new, evolving goals is crucial for ongoing growth. As you achieve one milestone, look for the next area to improve. These goals should align with your changing life circumstances and aspirations. For instance, if you've successfully managed emotional eating, you might set a new goal to enhance your physical fitness or improve your mental well-being. Identifying areas for further improvement keeps you focused and driven. It's not about perfection; it's about making steady progress and continually striving to be the best version of yourself.

Embracing a lifelong growth mindset means continually seeking new opportunities for learning and self-improvement. Staying informed through reading and research helps you stay updated on the latest insights and strategies for managing emotional eating. Attending workshops, seminars, or support groups provides valuable connections and practical advice. Setting new, evolving goals keeps you focused and motivated, ensuring that you're always working towards personal development.

In the context of continuous growth, it's essential to revisit and reassess your goals regularly. Life is dynamic, and your priorities may shift over time. What was once a primary focus may become less relevant as you achieve progress in other areas. Periodically evaluating your goals ensures they align with your current needs and aspirations. This practice of reassessment helps you stay on track and adapt to changing circumstances, fostering a sense of purpose and direction in your journey.

One effective strategy for ongoing growth is to create a personal development plan. This plan can outline your short-term and long-term goals and the steps you'll take to achieve them. It should include specific actions, timelines, and resources you'll need. Regularly reviewing and updating your plan keeps you accountable and provides a clear roadmap for your journey. This structured approach to personal development helps you stay organized and focused, making it easier to track your progress and celebrate your achievements.

Reflecting on and learning from your experiences is another crucial aspect of continuous growth. Each setback, challenge, or achievement offers valuable lessons. Take time to reflect on what worked well, what didn't, and how you can apply these insights moving forward. This reflective practice fosters a growth mindset, encouraging you to view each experience as an opportunity for learning and self-improvement. By embracing this mindset, you can navigate the ups and downs of your journey with resilience and optimism.

Embracing a lifelong growth mindset means recognizing that your journey is ongoing and ever-evolving. Setbacks are opportunities for learning, and each challenge you face is a chance to grow stronger. By staying informed, attending workshops, and setting new goals, you can continue to evolve and improve. Reflecting on your experiences and learning from them fosters resilience and optimism. Through continuous growth, you can build a healthier relationship with food and yourself, creating a fulfilling and balanced life.

CONCLUSION

As we end this journey together, I want to reflect on everything we've covered. From understanding the roots of emotional eating to identifying triggers, cultivating mindful eating practices, and building a toolbox of coping strategies, you've embarked on a path of self-discovery and growth. We've explored the role of self-compassion, the impact of society and media, and the importance of developing a holistic approach to well-being.

One of the key takeaways from this book is that emotional eating is not a matter of lock of willpower or discipline. It's a complex behavior rooted in our emotions, past experiences, and environment. By understanding these underlying factors, you can begin breaking the emotional eating cycle. Recognizing your triggers, whether they are emotional, environmental, or psychological, is the first step toward change. Remember, awareness is a powerful tool.

Mindful eating is another crucial lesson we've discussed. You can transform your relationship with food by bringing awareness and intention to your eating habits. Paying attention to hunger and fullness cues and eating without distractions can help you enjoy your meals and prevent overeating.

Self-compassion plays a vital role in this journey. Treating yourself with kindness and understanding can make a significant difference, especially during challenging times. Instead of criticizing yourself for setbacks, offer words of encouragement and support. Embracing imperfection and focusing on progress rather than perfection can help you build a positive self-image.

Creating a supportive environment at home and work can also make a significant impact. Surround yourself with healthy options, set up designated eating spaces, and seek support from friends, family, or professional help. Remember, you don't have to do this alone. Building a support network can provide the encouragement and accountability you need to stay on track.

As you continue on this journey, I want to empower you with some words of encouragement. Change is not easy, and it takes time. Be patient with yourself and celebrate every small victory along the way. No matter how small, each step you take is a step towards a healthier and more balanced life. Believe in your ability to overcome challenges and create lasting change.

Now, I encourage you to take action. Reflect on what you've learned and identify specific steps you can take to continue your progress. Maybe it's keeping a food diary, practicing mindful eating, or setting realistic goals. Perhaps it's reaching out to a friend or joining a support group. Whatever it is, take that first step today. Your journey doesn't end here; it's just beginning.

In closing, I want to leave you with a final motivational message. You are stronger and more resilient than you realize. The fact that you picked up this book and committed to this journey speaks volumes about your determination and courage. Remember, you have the power to create the life you want. Embrace the process, be kind to yourself, and keep moving forward. Your future is filled with possibilities, and I am confident you will achieve great things.

Thank you for allowing me to be a part of your journey. I am proud of the progress you've made and excited for the growth that lies ahead. Here's to a healthier, happier, and more balanced you!

REFERENCES

1. 3 CBT Techniques You Can Use Now for Disordered Eating. (n.d.). Retrieved from https://www.kindfulbody.com/3-cbt-techniques-you-can-use-now-for-disordered-eating
2. 6 Common Cognitive Distortions Behind Eating Disorders. (n.d.). Retrieved from https://www.centralcoasttreatmentcenter.com/blog-1/6-common-cognitive-distortions-behind-eating-disorders
3. 8 Powerful Self-Compassion Exercises & Worksheets. (n.d.). Retrieved from https://positivepsychology.com/self-compassion-exercises-worksheets
4. Body Image: What is it, and How Can I Improve It? (n.d.). Retrieved from https://www.medicalnewstoday.com/articles/249190
5. Brief Mindfulness Meditation Improves Emotion Processing. (n.d.). Retrieved from https://www.ncbi.nlm.nih.gov/pmc/articles/PMC6795685
6. Cognitive Behavioral Therapy for Eating Disorders. (n.d.). Retrieved from https://www.ncbi.nlm.nih.gov/pmc/articles/PMC2928448
7. Eating Disorder Support Groups. (n.d.). Retrieved from https://www.eatingrecoverycenter.com/support-groups
8. Eating Disorder Treatment and Recovery - HelpGuide.org. (n.d.). Retrieved from https://www.helpguide.org/articles/eating-disorders/eating-disorder-treatment-and-recovery
9. Emotional Eating and How to Stop It - HelpGuide.org. (n.d.). Retrieved from https://www.helpguide.org/articles/diets/emotional-eating
10. Emotional Eating: Why It Happens and How to Stop It. (n.d.). Retrieved from https://www.healthline.com/health/emotional-eating
11. Emotional Hunger vs. Physical Hunger: How to Tell The Difference. (n.d.). Retrieved from https://www.rachaelhartleynutrition.com/blog/emotional-hunger-vs-physical-hunger
12. Exercise for Mental Health. (n.d.). Retrieved from https://www.ncbi.nlm.nih.gov/pmc/articles/PMC1470658
13. Exploring the Meaning of Self-Compassion and Its Benefits. (n.d.). Retrieved from https://self-compassion.org/what-is-self-compassion
14. Food & Your Mood: How Food Affects Mental Health. (n.d.). Retrieved from https://www.aetna.com/health-guide/food-affects-mental-health
15. How To Start a Mindful Eating Practice - Mass General Hospital. (n.d.).

Retrieved from https://www.massgeneral.org/news/start-mindful-eating-practice
16. How to Prevent Emotional Eating Using Yoga. (n.d.). Retrieved from https://www.yogabasics.com/connect/yoga-blog/yoga-emotional-eating
17. Maslow's Hierarchy of Needs and Eating Disorder Recovery. (n.d.). Retrieved from https://sidebysidenutrition.com/blog/maslows
18. Media Literacy 10 Top Tips. (n.d.). Retrieved from https://www.bemediasmart.ie/tips/media-literacy-10-top-tips
19. Mindful Eating - The Nutrition Source. (n.d.). Retrieved from https://nutritionsource.hsph.harvard.edu/mindful-eating
20. Mindful Eating And Dancing Led To My 113-Lb. Weight Loss. (n.d.). Retrieved from https://www.womenshealthmag.com/weight-loss/a29953771/mindful-eating-weight-loss-success-story
21. Nutritional Psychiatry: Your Brain on Food. (n.d.). Retrieved from https://www.health.harvard.edu/blog/nutritional-psychiatry-your-brain-on-food-201511168626
22. Relationship Between Mental Health and Emotional Eating. (n.d.). Retrieved from https://www.ncbi.nlm.nih.gov/pmc/articles/PMC9573278
23. Role of Physical Activity on Mental Health and Well-Being. (n.d.). Retrieved from https://www.ncbi.nlm.nih.gov/pmc/articles/PMC9902068
24. Role of Sleep and Sleep Loss in Hormonal Release. (n.d.). Retrieved from https://www.ncbi.nlm.nih.gov/pmc/articles/PMC3065172
25. Self-Compassion Research by Kristin Neff. (n.d.). Retrieved from https://self-compassion.org/the-research
26. SMART Goals for Eating Disorder Recovery. (n.d.). Retrieved from https://evolvetherapy.org/smart-goals-for-eating-disorder-recovery
27. Stress and Emotional Eating - Leadership Skills & Stress Relief with Bosch Integrative Wellness. (n.d.). Retrieved from https://boschintegrativewellness.com/resiliency/emotional-eating
28. Stress, Cortisol, and Other Appetite-Related Hormones. (n.d.). Retrieved from https://www.ncbi.nlm.nih.gov/pmc/articles/PMC5373497
29. Success Stories. (n.d.). Retrieved from https://escapefromemotionaleating.com/success-stories
30. The Benefits of Food Journaling. (n.d.). Retrieved from https://www.beebehealthcare.org/health-hub/nutrition/benefits-food-journaling
31. The Harmful Effects of Diet Culture and Social Media. (n.d.). Retrieved from https://very.health/the-harmful-effects-of-diet-culture-and-social-media
32. The Importance of Celebrating Milestones. (n.d.). Retrieved from https://online.maryville.edu/blog/importance-of-celebrating-milestones
33. The History of the 'Ideal' Woman and Where That Has Left Us. (n.d.).

Retrieved from https://www.cnn.com/2018/03/07/health/body-image-history-of-beauty-explainer-intl/index.html

34. The Power of Self-Compassion - Harvard Health. (n.d.). Retrieved from https://www.health.harvard.edu/healthbeat/the-power-of-self-compassion
35. The Role of Emotion Processing in Art Therapy (REPAT). (n.d.). Retrieved from https://www.ncbi.nlm.nih.gov/pmc/articles/PMC10343444
36. Unlocking Motivational Blocks: Why is it so Hard to Make Changes in My Diet?. (n.d.). Retrieved from https://therawfoodkitchen.com/motivational-blocks-why-is-it-so-hard
37. Weight Loss: Gain Control of Emotional Eating - Mayo Clinic. (n.d.). Retrieved from https://www.mayoclinic.org/healthy-lifestyle/weight-loss/in-depth/weight-loss/art-20047342

ABOUT THE AUTHOR

Lawrence E. Meadows is the author of *Triumph Over Emotional Eating,* a guide to overcoming emotional eating challenges and building healthier relationships with food. Lawrence holds a degree in Behavioral Neuroscience, which has equipped him with deep insights into the mind-body connection and how emotions influence eating behaviors. His personal journey with emotional eating, combined with his academic background, inspired him to write this book to help others break free from unhealthy habits and develop mindful eating practices. Lawrence lives in the United States with his wife and two children, where he enjoys spending time with family and exploring the outdoors.

Printed in Great Britain
by Amazon

54342318R00086